Contents

Introduction

Welcome to the study of human disease. Your textbook, *An Introduction to Human Disease,* was based on courses given to undergraduate and graduate students like you who have mastered the essential concepts of human disease. Many have gone on to careers in biology, medicine, nursing, and other health fields. Each chapter in your book begins with learning objectives, followed by a systematic survey of the pathology, pathophysiology, clinical manifestations, and principles of treatment of the important diseases considered in each chapter. Each chapter then finishes with an annotated bibliography that points you toward important articles in the medical literature related to the subjects considered in the chapter.

This workbook will help you navigate through the course. It includes diagrams, Power-Point presentations, and various types of exercises to test and reinforce your comprehension of the essential features of the diseases you will be studying. To get you started on your journey of discovery, the workbook begins with a listing of the important points considered in the first five chapters of your book. You will build on these concepts as you continue into other chapters dealing with specific organ system derangements.

I believe that you will be pleasantly surprised to find that the basic concepts relating to human disease are quite straightforward, easy to understand, and extremely interesting. You have undoubtedly completed a course in anatomy and physiology, and you already know that every organ system has key structural features and physiologic functions. All is well when the systems function properly. When you know normal structure and function, it is not hard to understand what happens when systems don't function properly, producing disease. Moreover, when you understand the anatomic and physiologic changes associated with a disease, you can usually deduce the clinical manifestations of the disease, and can understand how treatment favorably influences its course and outcome.

The benefit you derive from the course will depend to a large extent on your own efforts. The course follows the class schedule closely. To get the most from the class, read over the material to be covered before you attend the lecture or classroom exercise so that you are familiar with what is to be covered. Then you will be in a better position to get more out of the lectures and other classroom activities dealing with the subjects considered in the assigned chapters. After the class, reread the material covered in class while the material is still fresh in your mind, and use the workbook material to help you. This approach will help you "nail down" your comprehension of the material. Such a systematic approach to learning the material will pay big dividends, and you will derive tremendous satisfaction from watching your knowledge base relating to human disease grow by "leaps and bounds" as you proceed through the course.

Enjoy your adventure. Have a pleasant journey.

Leonard Crowley

A ... n
to ... ase

Department of Laboratory Medicine and Pathology
University of Minnesota Medical School, Minneapolis

Professor
Biology Department
Century College

JONES AND BARTLETT PUBLISHERS
Sudbury, Massachusetts
BOSTON   TORONTO   LONDON   SINGAPORE

World Headquarters
Jones and Bartlett Publishers
40 Tall Pine Drive
Sudbury, MA 01776
978-443-5000
info@jbpub.com
www.jbpub.com

Jones and Bartlett Publishers Canada
2406 Nikanna Road
Mississauga, ON L5C 2W6
CANADA

Jones and Bartlett Publishers International
Barb House, Barb Mews
London W6 7PA
UK

Production Credits
Acquisitions Editor: Jacqueline Ann Mark
Senior Production Editor: Julie C. Bolduc
Associate Editor: Nicole Quinn
Editorial Assistant: Erin Murphy
Marketing Manager: Ed McKenna
Manufacturing Buyer: Therese Bräuer
Composition: Interactive Composition Corporation
Cover Design: Anne Spencer
Printing and Binding: Courier Stoughton
Cover Printing: Courier Stoughton

ISBN: 0-7637-2963-9

Printed in the United States of America
08 07 06 05 04   10 9 8 7 6 5 4 3 2

Chapter 1 General Concepts of Disease: Principles of Diagnosis

Chapter Outline

The chapter outline provides you with an organizational guide to the topics and ideas presented in this chapter of the text.

Characteristics of Disease
Classifications of Disease
    Congenital and Hereditary Diseases
    Inflammatory Diseases
    Degenerative Diseases
    Metabolic Diseases
    Neoplastic Diseases
Health and Disease: A Continuum
Principles of Diagnosis
    The History
    The Physical Examination
    Treatment
Screening Tests for Disease
    Purpose and Requirements for Effective Screening
    Groups Suitable for Screening
    Suitable Screening Tests
    Benefits of Screening
    Screening for Genetic Disease
Diagnostic Tests and Procedures
    Clinical Laboratory Tests
    Tests of Electrical Activity
    Radioisotope (Radionuclide) Studies
    Endoscopy
    Ultrasound
    X-Ray Examination
    Magnetic Resonance Imaging
    Positron Emission Tomography
    Cytologic and Histologic Examinations

Introductory Concepts in Chapter 1

The following material is provided as a guide to some of the fundamental concepts in the first five chapters. It may help you organize the material as you get started in this course. You will build upon these concepts as you begin to study diseases involving various organ systems.

1. Disease is a disturbance of the structure or function of the body.
2. Disease produces various manifestations: signs, symptoms, and abnormal laboratory test results.
3. The clinician's task is to determine the nature of the disease (make a diagnosis), estimate the probable outcome of the disease (prognosis), and then treat the patient (symptomatic and specific treatment).
4. Look over the various diagnostic procedures available to the physician, but learning the details of them is not necessary now.
5. We will talk about screening for disease in a population. Screening requires three things: a "screenable population" (significant frequency of disease); a reliable, cost-effective test to identify the disease that can be performed without risk to the patient; and evidence that early detection of the disease will favorably influence outcome.

Study Questions

The following questions are provided as a test for comprehension and as a study guide for use with the text chapters. Additional study material is located at http://health.jbpub.com/humandisease/, which contains useful eLearning tools such as an A&P review, animated flashcards, interactive online glossary, crossword puzzles, and Web links.

Key Terms

Define the following terms:

1. Etiology _____

2. Symptom of disease _____

3. Sign of disease _____

4. Diagnosis _____

5. Prognosis _____

6. Specific treatment _____

7. Symptomatic treatment _____

8. Pathogen _____

9. Pathogenesis _____

Fill-in-the-Blank

1. A test based on echoes produced in tissues by high-frequency sound waves is _____.

2. A young woman has a skin rash caused by an allergic reaction to an antibiotic. This patient's condition would be classified as _____.

3. The opinion of a physician concerning the eventual outcome of a disease in a patient is called _____.

4. A disease in which the principal manifestation is an abnormal growth of cells leading to formation of tumors is called _____.

Identify

1. Identify the five major categories of diseases, and indicate the characteristic features of each type.

   a. _____

   b. _____

   c. _____

   d. _____

   e. _____

2. Identify the nine major categories of diagnostic tests and procedures available to help the physician or other health practitioner diagnose and treat a patient properly.

   a. _____

   b. _____

   c. _____

   d. _____

e. _____

f. _____

g. _____

h. _____

i. _____

3. Identify the five major categories of human disease.

   a. _____

   b. _____

   c. _____

   d. _____

   e. _____

4. Identify three tests that measure the electrical impulses associated with various body functions and activities.

   a. _____

   b. _____

   c. _____

5. Identify the tests or procedures that would be useful to assist the physician in evaluating the following conditions in a patient.

   a. Urinary tract infection _____

   b. Fractured wrist _____

   c. Possible "heart attack" _____

   d. A lump in the breast _____

   e. Amenorrhea in a young woman _____

   f. The maturity of a fetus and the location of the placenta within the mother's uterus _____

   _____

Discussion Questions

1. Describe the differences between a diagnosis and a prognosis. _____

   _____

   _____

   _____

2. Describe the steps a physician or other health practitioner uses to make a diagnosis of a specific disease or condition in a patient. _____

   _____

   _____

   _____

3. What is the difference between symptomatic treatment and specific treatment? _____

_____

_____

_____

4. You wish to develop a program to screen for a specific disease, such as diabetes. Describe the requirements for a successful screening program. _____

_____

_____

_____

5. A middle-aged man consults his physician because of cough, fever, chest pain, and purulent sputum. What diagnostic measures will assist the physician in determining the cause of the patient's illness? _____

_____

_____

_____

6. A governmental agency proposes a pilot program to screen a population for a disease by means of a blood test. The characteristics of the disease and the screening test are listed here. Which of these characteristics indicate that the proposed screen is likely to be worthwhile, and which indicate that it is likely not to be worthwhile? Explain your answers.

   a. The disease occurs with some frequency (1 per 1000 persons screened).

   _____

   b. The disease progresses slowly in affected persons.

   _____

   c. No specific method of treatment is available at the present time.

   _____

   d. The test can detect the disease in its early stage and is relatively inexpensive (about $42.50).

   _____

   e. The test is quite specific, producing few false-positive or false-negative results.

   _____

7. A patient has a chronic cough, fever, and purulent sputum, and a lung infection (pneumonia) is suspected. What diagnostic procedures are likely to provide useful information? _____

_____

_____

_____

DISEASE

FUNCTIONAL
ORGANIC = LESIONS

MANIFESTATIONS
- SYMPTOMS
- SIGNS (PHYSICAL FINDINGS)
- ABNORMAL "LABORATORY" TESTS

TERMS
DIAGNOSIS - PROGNOSIS - TREATMENT
    PATHOGENESIS - LESION

A SYMPTOMATIC
SYMPTOMATIC

CLASSIFICATION

CONGENITAL
INFLAMMATORY
DEGENERATIVE
METABOLIC
NEOPLASTIC

SCREENING TESTS TO DETECT DISEASE

REQUIREMENTS

1. "SCREENABLE" POPULATION

2. RELIABLE COST EFFECTIVE TEST WITHOUT RISK TO SUBJECT

3. EARLY DETECTION OF DISEASE WILL FAVORABLY INFLUENCE OUTCOME

Notes

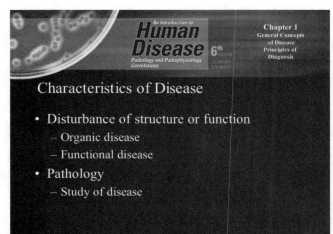

Characteristics of Disease

- Disturbance of structure or function
  - Organic disease
  - Functional disease
- Pathology
  - Study of disease

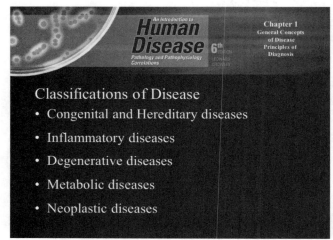

Classifications of Disease
- Congenital and Hereditary diseases
- Inflammatory diseases
- Degenerative diseases
- Metabolic diseases
- Neoplastic diseases

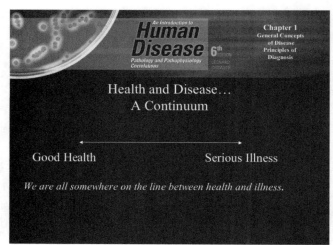

Health and Disease...
A Continuum

Good Health   Serious Illness

We are all somewhere on the line between health and illness.

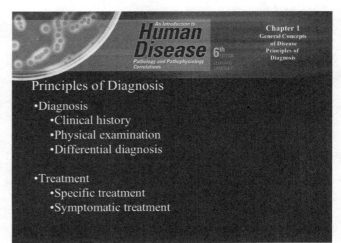

Principles of Diagnosis

- Diagnosis
  - Clinical history
  - Physical examination
  - Differential diagnosis

- Treatment
  - Specific treatment
  - Symptomatic treatment

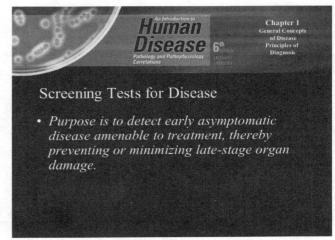

Screening Tests for Disease

- *Purpose is to detect early asymptomatic disease amenable to treatment, thereby preventing or minimizing late-stage organ damage.*

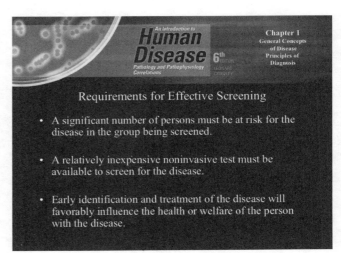

Requirements for Effective Screening

- A significant number of persons must be at risk for the disease in the group being screened.

- A relatively inexpensive noninvasive test must be available to screen for the disease.

- Early identification and treatment of the disease will favorably influence the health or welfare of the person with the disease.

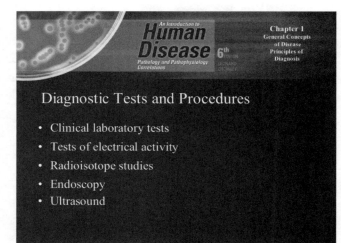

Diagnostic Tests and Procedures

- Clinical laboratory tests
- Tests of electrical activity
- Radioisotope studies
- Endoscopy
- Ultrasound

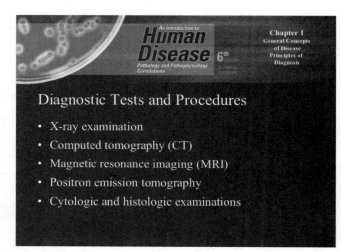

Diagnostic Tests and Procedures

- X-ray examination
- Computed tomography (CT)
- Magnetic resonance imaging (MRI)
- Positron emission tomography
- Cytologic and histologic examinations

Chapter Outline

The chapter outline provides you with an organizational guide to the topics and ideas presented in this chapter of the text.

Organization of Cells
The Cell
  The Nucleus
  The Cytoplasm
Tissues
  Epithelium
  Connective and Supporting Tissues
  Muscle Tissue
  Nerve Tissue
Organs and Organ Systems
The Germ Layers and Their Derivatives
Cell Function and the Genetic Code
  The Structure of DNA
  Duplication (Replication) of DNA
  The Genetic Code
Movement of Materials into and out of Cells
  Diffusion and Osmosis
  Active Transport
  Phagocytosis and Pinocytosis
Adaptations of Cells to Changing Conditions
  Atrophy
  Hypertrophy and Hyperplasia
  Metaplasia
  Dysplasia
  Increased Enzyme Synthesis
Cell Injury, Cell Death, and Cell Necrosis
  Cell Injury
  Cell Death and Cell Necrosis
  Programmed Cell Death: Apoptosis
Aging and the Cell

Introductory Concepts in Chapter 2

The following material is provided as a guide to some of the fundamental concepts in the first five chapters. It may help you organize the material as you get started in this course. You will build upon these concepts as you begin to study diseases involving various organ systems.

1. The cell is the basic structural and functional unit of the body. All cells have similar features (nucleus, cytoplasm, organelles), but many cells are specialized to perform specific functions.
2. The nucleus contains the genetic material (23 pairs of chromosomes = the genome) that directs the functions of the cell (via messenger RNA). The cytoplasm contains the various organelles (e.g., mitochondria, ribosomes, endoplasmic reticulum, lysosomes) that carry out the functions specified by DNA (see Fig. 2-8).
3. Groups of similar cells form tissues. Tissues are organized to form organs, and groups of organs form organ systems.

4. Epithelium covers the exterior of the body, lines the interior of organs such as the respiratory and GI tracts, lines body cavities, forms glands, and forms the functional cells of organs that have excretory or secretory functions (such as the liver and kidneys). Epithelium is classified on the basis of its structure (simple or stratified; squamous, transitional, or columnar). Connective tissue connects and supports. Muscle contracts, and nerve tissue conducts.

5. Materials move in and out of cells across cell membranes by active transport, phagocytosis, and pinocytosis (active processes that require the cell to expend energy), and by diffusion and osmosis (passive, non-energy-requiring processes).

6. Cells adapt to changing conditions (atrophy, hypertrophy, hyperplasia, metaplasia, dysplasia, increased enzyme synthesis).

7. Injured cells exhibit structural and functional abnormalities—swelling, fatty change, and necrosis, for example.

8. Normal cells don't last forever. They have a predetermined life span, and they wear out. (As we will see later, some tumor cells can proliferate indefinitely. They are "immortal.")

Study Questions

The following questions are provided as a test for comprehension and as a study guide for use with the text chapter. Additional study material is located at http://health.jbpub.com/humandisease/, which contains useful eLearning tools such as an A&P review, animated flashcards, interactive online glossary, crossword puzzles, and Web links.

Key Terms

Define the following terms:

1. Genetic code _____

2. Organelle _____

3. Hyperplasia _____

4. Dysplasia _____

5. Osmosis _____

6. Diffusion _____

7. Metaplasia _____

True/False

Tell whether each statement is true or false. If false, explain why the statement is incorrect.

1. The nucleus directs the metabolic functions of the cell. _____

   _____

2. Organelles are small chromosome fragments present in the nucleus. _____

   _____

3. Lysosomes digest material brought into the cell by phagocytosis. _____

   _____

4. All cells survive the same length of time within the body. _____

   _____

5. Migration of water molecules from a more dilute solution to a more concentrated solution across the semipermeable membrane is called diffusion. _____

   _____

Identify

1. Identify eight components within a typical cell and indicate the function of each.

   a. _____

   b. _____

   c. _____

   d. _____

e. _____

f. _____

g. _____

h. _____

2. Identify the four major types of tissues and briefly describe the functions of each type.

a. _____

b. _____

c. _____

d. _____

3. Identify the three germ layers that develop from the fertilized ovum, and indicate what structures develop from each layer. (*Hint:* See Fig. 2-5.)

a. _____

b. _____

c. _____

4. Identify the five ways in which cells adapt to changing conditions.

a. _____

b. _____

c. _____

d. _____

e. _____

Discussion Questions

1. Diagram the structure of a typical cell. Indicate the functions of the major organelles.

2. What is the difference between cell hyperplasia and dysplasia? _____

_____

_____

_____

3. How does the cell respond to injury? _____

_____

_____

_____

4. What are the major difference between epithelium and connective tissue? _____

_____

_____

_____

5. Briefly describe the structures and main functions of the various types of epithelium. _____

_____

_____

_____

6. List and describe the various ways that materials move in and out of cells across the cell membrane. _____

_____

_____

_____

7. Describe how osmosis differs from diffusion. _____

_____

_____

_____

8. Describe the difference between cell metaplasia and cell dysplasia. _____

_____

_____

_____

9. Describe some of the important changes that occur in an aging cell, and describe ways by which we can retard aging changes in cells. _____

_____

_____

_____

THE CELL

Components
- _Nucleus_: Genetic Material
- _Cytoplasm_: Organelles
  - Mitochondria
  - Endoplasmic Reticulum: Smooth / Rough
  - Golgi Apparatus
  - Lysosomes
  - Centrioles
  - Cytoskeleton: Filaments and Tubules

Movement of Material in and out of Cells
- _Passive_: with Concentration Gradient
  - Dissolved Materials: Diffusion
  - Water: Osmosis
- _Active Transport_: Against Concentration Gradient
- _Engulfed_: Phagocytosis / Pinocytosis

Cell Adaptations
- Atrophy : Decrease Size
- Hypertrophy: Increase Size
- Hyperplasia: More Cells
- Metaplasia : Changed Cell, Adaptation
- Dysplasia : Disorderly Change
- Neoplasia. Tumor

Cell Injury
- _Cell Swelling_: Impaired Na/K Transport
  - Na Diffuses into Cell with Water
- _Fatty Change_: Impaired Fat Metabolism

Cell Death: (Structural Change: Necrosis)

Cell Aging:
- Predetermined Life Span
- Environmental Agents Damage DNA/RNA Organelles
- Ability to Repair Damage Affects Survival

TISSUES

EPITHELIUM: LINES, COVERS, FUNCTIONAL CELLS OF GLANDS / ORGANS WITH EXCRETORY / SECRETORY FUNCTION
- FLAT PLATES
- CUBES
- COLUMNS
- "SQUASHED" COLUMNS
} DIFFERENTIAL FEATURES

MESOTHELIUM

ENDOTHELIUM

MEMBRANES
- EPITHELIAL
- SEROUS
- MUCOUS

CONNECTIVE / SUPPORTING
- SYNOVIAL MEMBRANES

MUSCLE

NERVE

Notes

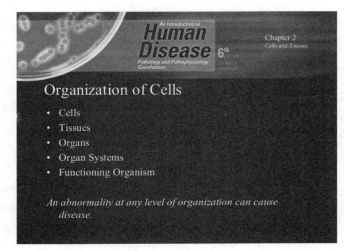

Organization of Cells

- Cells
- Tissues
- Organs
- Organ Systems
- Functioning Organism

An abnormality at any level of organization can cause disease.

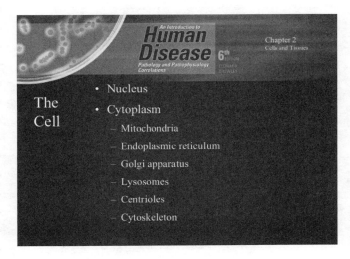

The Cell

- Nucleus
- Cytoplasm
  - Mitochondria
  - Endoplasmic reticulum
  - Golgi apparatus
  - Lysosomes
  - Centrioles
  - Cytoskeleton

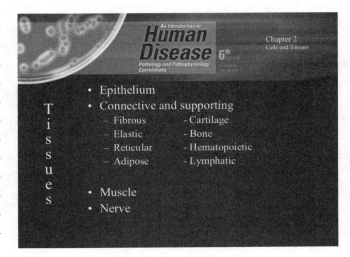

Tissues

- Epithelium
- Connective and supporting
  - Fibrous   - Cartilage
  - Elastic   - Bone
  - Reticular   - Hematopoietic
  - Adipose   - Lymphatic
- Muscle
- Nerve

Notes

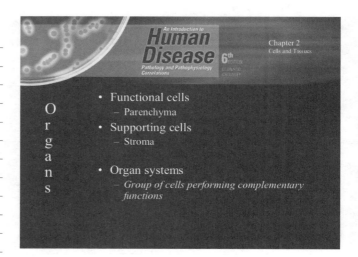

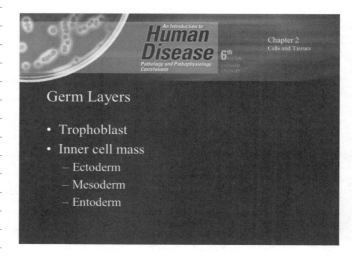

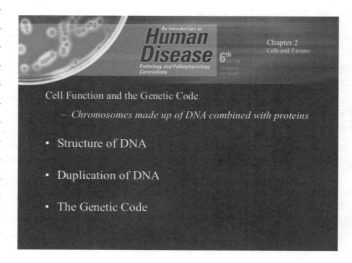

Notes

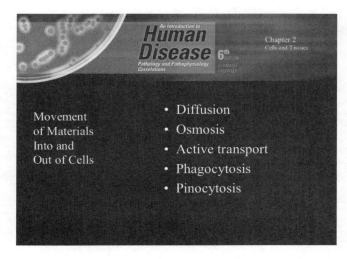

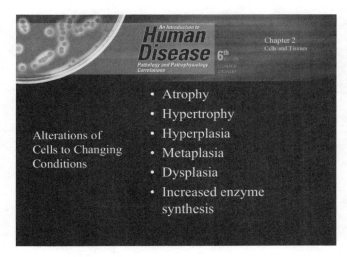

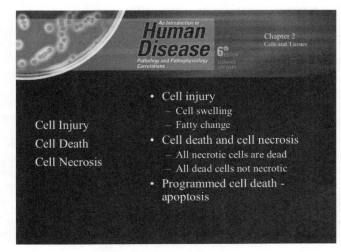

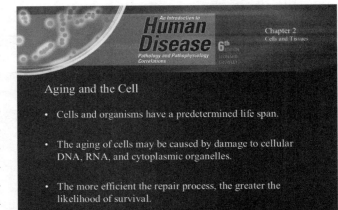

Aging and the Cell

- Cells and organisms have a predetermined life span.

- The aging of cells may be caused by damage to cellular DNA, RNA, and cytoplasmic organelles.

- The more efficient the repair process, the greater the likelihood of survival.

Chapter 3   Chromosomes, Genes, and Cell Division

Chapter Outline

The chapter outline provides you with an organizational guide to the topics and ideas presented in this chapter of the text.

Chromosomes
    Sex Chromosomes
Cell Division
    Mitosis
    Meiosis
Gametogenesis
    Spermatogenesis
    Oogenesis
    Comparison of Spermatogenesis and Oogenesis
Chromosome Analysis
Genes and Inheritance
    Gene Imprinting
    Mitochondrial Genes and Inheritance
Genes of the Histocompatibility (HLA) Complex
    HLA Types and Susceptibility to Disease
Genes and Recombinant DNA Technology (Genetic Engineering)
Gene Therapy

Introductory Concepts in Chapter 3

The following material is provided as a guide to some of the fundamental concepts in the first five chapters. It may help you organize the material as you get started in this course. You will build upon these concepts as you begin to study diseases involving various organ systems.

1. Chromosomes occur in pairs: 22 matched pairs of homologous chromosomes called autosomes (non-sex chromosomes) and one pair of sex chromosomes (XX = females; XY = male). One member of each chromosome pair comes from each parent.

2. Genes occupy specific sites on chromosomes called *gene loci*. There are paired gene loci on the paired chromosomes. At any gene locus, any one of several related genes can occupy the locus. These alternative forms of genes are called *alleles* or *allelic genes*. A person is homozygous for a gene if both gene loci possess the same allelic gene; a person is heterozygous if the alleles are different. See the text for descriptions of dominant, recessive, codominant, and sex-linked genes and their effects.

3. There are two types of cell division: *mitosis,* characteristic of somatic cells, and *meiosis,* which occurs in germ cells. Each cell has already duplicated its DNA before it ever starts to divide.

4. Mitosis is simply a separation of already duplicated chromosomes. Each precursor (parent) cell produces two daughter cells, each one identical to the parent cell.

5. Meiosis is a two-phase process. In the *first division,* some intermixing of genetic material between homologous chromosomes occurs, and then the chromosomes separate without dividing. Each parent cell produces two daughter cells, each having only one member of each homologous pair of chromosomes (these homologous chromosomes are slightly different than those in the parents because of the intermixing of genetic material between homologous chromosomes). The *second division* is just like mitosis, but only 23 chromosomes separate. Each of the daughter cells from the first division, in turn, gives rise to two more daughter cells. The final result is that each precursor cell eventually gives rise to daughter cells in two divisions.

6. See the text for a description of the differences between spermatogenesis and oogenesis. These differences will be important when we consider chromosomal abnormalities such as Down syndrome.

7. The HLA (MHC) system is a system of interconnected (linked) genes located at gene loci on one pair of homologous chromosomes that determine specific proteins (self-antigens) called HLA or MHC proteins on the surface of cells. The HLA genes are transmitted in sets called *haplotypes,* with one set being provided by each parent (see Fig. 3-9). There are multiple possible alleles at each gene locus, and there are so many possible gene combinations that each individual has a unique set of HLA antigens (except identical twins, who possess identical genes). Certain HLA types appear to be associated with increased susceptibility to certain diseases.

Study Questions

The following questions are provided as a test for comprehension and as a study guide for use with the text chapters. Additional study material is located at http://health.jbpub.com/humandisease/, which contains useful eLearning tools such as an A&P review, animated flashcards, interactive online glossary, crossword puzzles, and Web links.

Key Terms

Define the following terms:

1. Allele _____

2. Dominant gene _____

3. Recessive gene _____

4. Homozygous _____

5. Heterozygous _____

6. Hemizygous _____

7. Human leukocyte antigen (HLA) _____

8. Haplotype _____

9. Gene therapy _____

True/False

Tell whether each statement is true or false. If false, explain why the statement is incorrect.

1. The human genome consists of about 3 billion pairs of DNA bases, and most of the DNA on chromosomes consists of genes that regulate cell structure and functions. _____

   _____

2. The Human Genome Project has identified all of the genes on the human chromosomes and has determined the function of each of these genes. _____

   _____

3. Minor variations in the sequence of the nucleotides within the same genes of different individuals (gene polymorphism) may lead to differences in the way the genes are expressed. _____

   _____

4. A gene inherited from a female parent does not always have the same effect as the identical gene inherited from the male parent. _____

   _____

5. Chromosomes normally exist in pairs called homologous chromosomes. _____

   _____

6. Certain HLA types appear to predispose a person to specific diseases. _____

   _____

7. Genes exist in pairs, and the members of each pair are located at corresponding sites (gene loci) on homologous chromosomes. _____

_____

8. An individual is heterozygous for a gene if the genes at the corresponding loci on homologous chromosomes are the same, and homozygous for the gene if the genes are different. _____

_____

9. A dominant gene expresses itself in either the homozygous or heterozygous state. _____

_____

10. An X-linked gene is one that occurs *only* in the female. _____

_____

11. A defective X-linked gene may not cause clinical manifestations in the female, but may be associated with major clinical manifestations in the male. _____

_____

12. Tell whether each of the following statements regarding identification of inherited disease in newborn infants by screening tests is true or false. If false, explain why the statement is incorrect.

   a. Screening is unlikely to be useful because most inherited diseases do not respond to treatment. _____

   _____

   b. Long-term harmful effects of inherited diseases can often be prevented by early treatment. _____

   _____

   c. Identification of a hereditary disease in a newborn may allow parents to make an informed decision regarding future pregnancies, based on the nature of the inherited disease and its prognosis. _____

   _____

Discussion Questions

1. Describe the major differences between mitosis and meiosis. _____

_____

_____

_____

2. Describe how spermatogenesis differs from oogenesis. _____

_____

_____

_____

3. What is the Human Genome Project? _____

_____

_____

_____

4. Describe the Lyon hypothesis relating to X chromosome inactivation. _____

_____

_____

_____

5. What is a karyotype? How is it determined? _____

_____

_____

_____

6. Describe what goals must be achieved for gene therapy to be successful. _____

_____

_____

_____

GENES, CHROMOSOMES, CELL DIVISION

GENES   SEGMENT OF DNA CHAIN THAT
DIRECTS SYNTHESIS OF A PROTEIN
(GENE PRODUCT)
ARRANGED ON CHROMOSOME "LIKE
BEADS ON A STRING"

CHROMOSOMES : 22 PAIR OF AUTOSOMES
     1 PAIR SEX CHROMOSOMES
ONLY ONE X IS REQUIRED FOR
NORMAL CELL FUNCTION EXCEPT VERY
EARLY IN EMBRYONIC DEVELOPMENT
THE OTHER X IN FEMALE IS INACTIVATED
AS <u>SEX CHROMATIN (BARR) BODY</u>.

GENE CONCEPTS:
<u>HOMOLOGOUS CHROMOSOMES PAIRED</u>
<u>GENES PAIRED AT CORRESPONDING POSITIONS</u>
<u>(LOCI) ON HOMOLOGOUS CHROMOSOMES</u>
<u>CONCEPT OF ALLELIC GENES</u>
<u>GENE EXPRESSION</u>
- **DOMINANT**: EXPRESSED IN HETEROZYGOTE
- **RECESSIVE**: EXPRESSED ONLY IN HOMOZYGOTE
- **CODOMINANT**: BOTH ALLELES EXPRESSED
- **X LINKED**: EXPRESSION DEPENDS ON
WHETHER PAIRED WITH ANOTHER X (IN FEMALE)
OR WITH Y (IN MALE)

CHROMOSOMES ARE DUPLICATED PRIOR
TO CELL DIVISION

ORIGINAL CHROMOSOMES AND DUPLICATED
COUNTERPARTS REMAIN ATTACHED AT
CENTROMERES

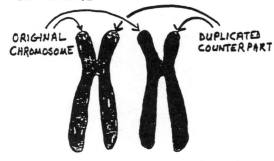

ONE PAIR OF HOMOLOGOUS CHROMOSOMES
THE JOINED ORIGINAL AND DUPLICATE ARE
CALLED CHROMATIDS

MITOSIS

CHROMATIDS SEPARATE AND TWO
IDENTICAL "DAUGHTER CELLS" FORM
FROM "PARENT CELL".

MEIOSIS

HOMOLOGOUS CHROMOSOMES JOIN AND
EXCHANGE SEGMENTS

THEN THEY SEPARATE, AND ONE
MEMBER OF PAIR GOES TO EACH
DAUGHTER CELL. CHROMOSOMES
REDUCED BY ONE HALF.

THEN EACH OF THE TWO DAUGHTER
CELLS DIVIDES, JUST LIKE MITOSIS.
CHROMATIDS SEPARATE.

EACH OF THE TWO DAUGHTER
CELLS FORMS TWO DAUGHTER CELLS.

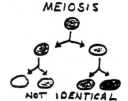

HLA (MHC) SYSTEM

A LINKED GENE SYSTEM DETERMINES
PROTEINS (ANTIGENS) ON CELLS.

<u>FOUR SEPARATE GENE LOCI</u> (A, B, C, D) ON
PAIRED CHROMOSOMES ARE TRANSMITTED AS
SETS (HAPLOTYPES). <u>MULTIPLE ALLELES</u> AT
EACH LOCUS

CHROMOSOME
CONTRIBUTED
BY MOTHER
BY FATHER

POSSIBLE ALLELES
A LOCUS > 45
B LOCUS > 50
C LOCUS > 11
D LOCUS > 50

OUR OWN HLA ANTIGENS NORMALLY DO
<u>NOT STIMULATE AN IMMUNE RESPONSE</u>.
THEY <u>ARE SELF-ANTIGENS</u> AND OUR IMMUNE
SYSTEM IS USED TO THEM.

BUT <u>THEY ARE FOREIGN ANTIGENS IN
OTHER PEOPLE</u> WHO HAVE DIFFERENT HLA
ANTIGENS, AND THE IMMUNE SYSTEM
DESTROYS THE CELLS WITH THE FOREIGN HLA
ANTIGENS.

Notes

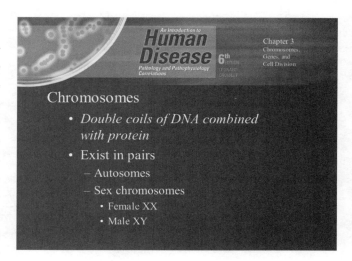

Chromosomes
- *Double coils of DNA combined with protein*
- Exist in pairs
  - Autosomes
  - Sex chromosomes
    - Female XX
    - Male XY

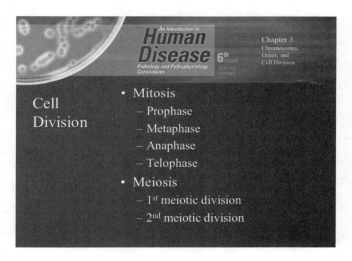

Cell Division
- Mitosis
  - Prophase
  - Metaphase
  - Anaphase
  - Telophase
- Meiosis
  - 1st meiotic division
  - 2nd meiotic division

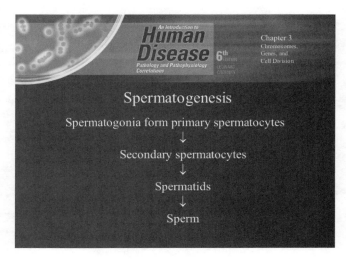

Spermatogenesis

Spermatogonia form primary spermatocytes
↓
Secondary spermatocytes
↓
Spermatids
↓
Sperm

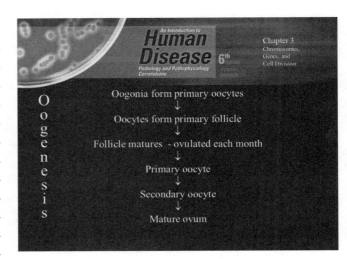

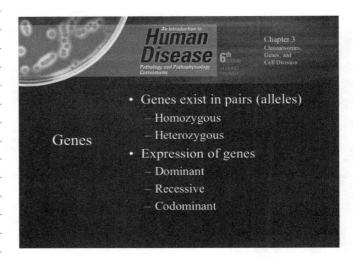

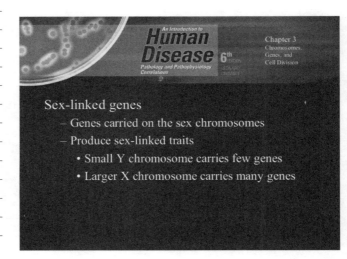

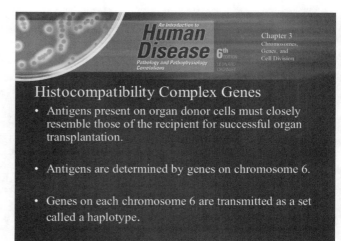

Histocompatibility Complex Genes

- Antigens present on organ donor cells must closely resemble those of the recipient for successful organ transplantation.

- Antigens are determined by genes on chromosome 6.

- Genes on each chromosome 6 are transmitted as a set called a haplotype.

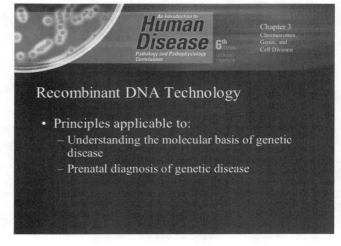

Recombinant DNA Technology

- Principles applicable to:
  - Understanding the molecular basis of genetic disease
  - Prenatal diagnosis of genetic disease

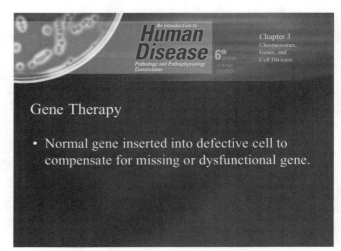

Gene Therapy

- Normal gene inserted into defective cell to compensate for missing or dysfunctional gene.

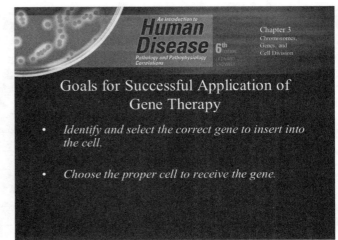

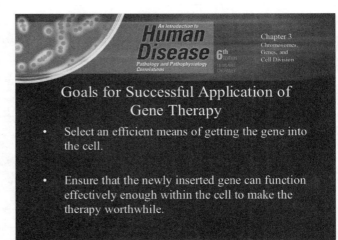

Chapter 4   Inflammation and Repair

Chapter Outline

The chapter outline provides you with an organizational guide to the topics and ideas presented in this chapter of the text.

The Inflammatory Reaction
    Chemical Mediators of Inflammation
    The Role of Lysosomal Enzymes in the Inflammatory Process
    Inflammation Caused by Antigen–Antibody Interaction
    Harmful Effects of Inflammation
Infection
    Terminology of Infection
    Factors Influencing the Outcome of an Infection

Introductory Concepts in Chapter 4

The following material is provided as a guide to some of the fundamental concepts in the first five chapters. It may help you organize the material as you get started in this course. You will build upon these concepts as you begin to study diseases involving various organ systems.

1. The inflammatory reaction is a nonspecific stereotyped response to cell injury. The response is always the same because any tissue injury triggers the release of the same type of mediators of inflammation (see Fig. 4-1). Mediators come from *mast cells* (mostly histamine), *platelets* (serotonin), and *other injured cells* (prostaglandins, leukotrienes); they also come from blood plasma (bradykinins) and from activation of blood proteins called *complement*.
2. Lysosomes (packs of digestive enzymes in the cytoplasm of white cells) release their digestive enzymes when white cells degenerate at the site of inflammation. The released lysosmal enzymes then cause further tissue injury.
3. Sometimes the tissue injury caused by the inflammation is so marked that it is necessary to suppress the inflammatory process by means of corticosteroids (such as cortisone) or nonsteroidal anti-inflammatory drugs (such as aspirin or ibuprofen).
4. Inflammation is a general term. If the inflammation is caused by a pathogenic microorganism, we use the term *infection*. Various terms are used to describe an infection: *cellulitis* (localized infection in the tissues), *lymphangitis* (infection spreading into lymphatic channels draining the site of infection, with red streaks running up the arm), *lymphadenitis* (regional lymph nodes involved), *abscess* (necrosis of tissue with a pocket of pus), and *septicemia* (bloodstream infection).
5. The outcome of an infection depends on whether the pathogen or body defenses win, or whether they are evenly matched and a chronic infection results (see Fig. 4-14).

Study Questions

The following questions are provided as a test for comprehension and as a study guide for use with the text chapters. Additional study material is located at http://health.jbpub.com/humandisease/, which contains useful eLearning tools such as an A&P review, animated flashcards, interactive online glossary, crossword puzzles, and Web links.

Key Terms

Define the following terms:

1. Exudate _____

2. Infection _____

3. Inflammation _____

4. Leukocytes _____

5. Pathogenic _____

6. Plasma _____

7. Lymphadenitis _____

8. Septicemia _____

9. Antibodies _____

10. Mediators of inflammation _____

11. Phagocytosis _____

12. Fibrinogen _____

13. Lysosome _____

Fill-in-the-Blank

1. _____ is a specialized connective-tissue cell containing granules filled with histamine and other chemical mediators.

2. A platelet is a component of the blood—a roughly circular or oval disk concerned with _____.

3. Serotonin is a _____ mediator of inflammation released from platelets.

4. _____ is a prostaglandinlike mediator of inflammation.

5. Bradykinin is a chemical mediator of inflammation derived from components in the _____.

6. _____ is an acute spreading inflammation affecting the skin or deeper tissues.

7. Lymphangitis is an inflammation of _____ draining a site of infection.

8. _____ is an infection in which large numbers of pathogenic bacteria are present in the bloodstream.

True/False

Tell whether each statement is true or false. If false, explain why the statement is incorrect.

1. Mediators of inflammation are produced primarily by neutrophils. _____

_____

2. The inflammatory reaction is a nonspecific response to any agent that injures cells. _____

_____

3. The inflammatory reaction concentrates leukocytes and antibodies at the site of inflammation. _____

_____

4. The plasma cell is the most important cell in acute inflammatory reaction. _____

_____

5. Lymphocytes phagocytize debris produced by the inflammatory process. _____

_____

6. A serous exudate resulting from an inflammation is yellow because it consists primarily of inflammatory cells.

_____

7. A fibrinous exudate is rich in fibrinogen, which coagulates to form fibrin and create a sticky film on the surface of
the inflamed tissue. _____

_____

8. Extensive destruction of tissue secondary to inflammation is often followed by scarring. _____

_____

Discussion Questions

1. What is the inflammatory reaction? Describe its clinical manifestations. (*Hint:* See Fig. 4-1.) _____

_____

_____

_____

2. What are mediators of inflammation? _____

_____

_____

_____

3. What is the source of the mediators of inflammation? _____

_____

_____

_____

4. Describe what part lysosomal enzymes play in perpetuating and intensifying the inflammatory reaction. _____

_____

_____

_____

5. What is the difference between the terms "infection" and "inflammation"? _____

_____

_____

_____

6. What factors influence the outcome of an infection? (*Hint:* See Fig. 4-14.) _____

_____

_____

_____

7. List the possible outcomes of an inflammation produced by a pathogenic bacteria. _____

_____

_____

_____

8. What is the difference between serous and fibrinous exudates? _____

_____

_____

_____

INFLAMMATION: A REACTION TO INJURY

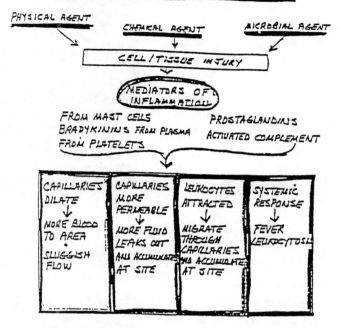

PHYSICAL AGENT   CHEMICAL AGENT   MICROBIAL AGENT

CELL / TISSUE INJURY

MEDIATORS OF INFLAMMATION

FROM MAST CELLS   PROSTAGLANDINS
BRADYKININS FROM PLASMA   ACTIVATED COMPLEMENT
FROM PLATELETS

CAPILLARIES DILATE	CAPILLARIES MORE PERMEABLE	LEUKOCYTES ATTRACTED	SYSTEMIC RESPONSE
↓ MORE BLOOD TO AREA • SLUGGISH FLOW	↓ MORE FLUID LEAKS OUT AND ACCUMULATES AT SITE	↓ MIGRATE THROUGH CAPILLARIES AND ACCUMULATE AT SITE	↓ FEVER LEUKOCYTOSIS

INFECTION = INFLAMMATION
CAUSED BY PATHOGENS

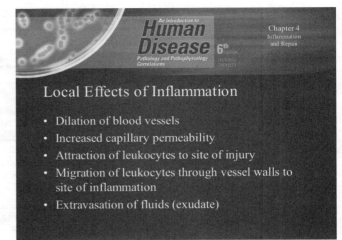

Local Effects of Inflammation

- Dilation of blood vessels
- Increased capillary permeability
- Attraction of leukocytes to site of injury
- Migration of leukocytes through vessel walls to site of inflammation
- Extravasation of fluids (exudate)

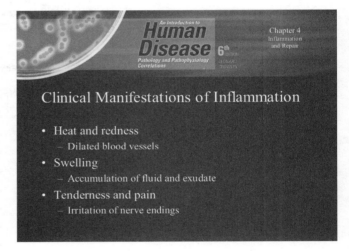

Clinical Manifestations of Inflammation

- Heat and redness
  - Dilated blood vessels
- Swelling
  - Accumulation of fluid and exudate
- Tenderness and pain
  - Irritation of nerve endings

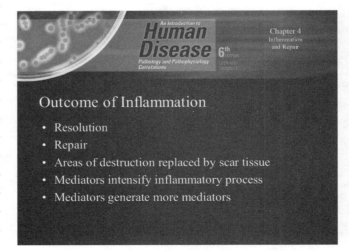

Outcome of Inflammation

- Resolution
- Repair
- Areas of destruction replaced by scar tissue
- Mediators intensify inflammatory process
- Mediators generate more mediators

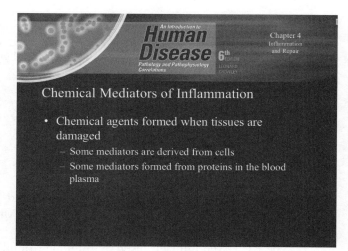

Chemical Mediators of Inflammation

- Chemical agents formed when tissues are damaged
  - Some mediators are derived from cells
  - Some mediators formed from proteins in the blood plasma

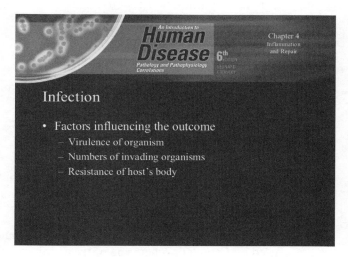

Infection

- Factors influencing the outcome
  - Virulence of organism
  - Numbers of invading organisms
  - Resistance of host's body

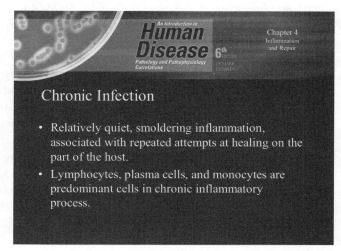

Chronic Infection

- Relatively quiet, smoldering inflammation, associated with repeated attempts at healing on the part of the host.
- Lymphocytes, plasma cells, and monocytes are predominant cells in chronic inflammatory process.

Chapter 5   Immunity, Hypersensitivity, Allergy, and Autoimmune Diseases

Chapter Outline

The chapter outline provides you with an organizational guide to the topics and ideas presented in this chapter of the text.

The Body's Defense Mechanisms
Immunity
    The Role of Lymphocytes in Acquired Immunity
    Development of the Lymphatic System
    Response of Lymphocytes to Foreign Antigens
    The Role of Complement in Immune Responses
Antibodies (Immunoglobulins)
Hypersensitivity Reactions: Immune System-Related Tissue Injury
    Type I. Immediate Hypersensitivity Reactions: Allergy and Anaphylaxis
    Type II. Cytotoxic Hypersensitivity Reactions
    Type III. Tissue Injury Caused by Immune Complexes ("Immune Complex Disease")
    Type IV. Delayed (Cell-Mediated) Hypersensitivity Reactions
Suppression of the Immune Response
    Reasons for Suppression
    Methods of Suppression
    Tissue Grafts and Immunity
Autoimmune Diseases
    Autoimmune Disease Manifestations and Mechanisms of Tissue Injury
    Connective-Tissue (Collagen) Diseases
    Lupus Erythematosus

Introductory Concepts in Chapter 5

The following material is provided as a guide to some of the fundamental concepts in the first five chapters. It may help you organize the material as you get started in this course. You will build upon these concepts as you begin to study diseases involving various organ systems.

1. Inflammation caused by a pathogenic microorganism (infection) differs from other types of inflammation caused by trauma or other type of tissue injury because the pathogen that causes the tissue injury is a *foreign substance* (non-self-antigen) that is introduced into the body. The body responds to its presence by generating an *immune response* to eliminate the foreign material in addition to giving rise to an inflammation.

2. The immune response may be *cell mediated* or *humoral*. Cell-mediated immunity is a property of T lymphocytes, which proliferate and accumulate around the foreign material, where they secrete destructive proteins called lymphokines. This is the main defense against viruses, fungi, parasites, and some bacteria such as the tubercle bacillus. Humoral immunity is a property of B lymphocytes. When stimulated by foreign material, they proliferate and "gear up" to produce large amounts of antibodies, which then combine with the foreign material. As B lymphocytes proliferate, they become transformed into cells with more cytoplasm that contains lots of ribosomes and rough endoplasmic reticulum. These cells are now called *plasma cells* and are very efficient "antibody-producing factories." This is our primary defense against most bacteria and bacterial toxins.

3. Several classes and types of antibodies (immunoglobulins) exist. See the fork analogy in the text on pages 88–89. IgM, a large molecule, is the first antibody formed. IgG (gamma globulin) is formed soon thereafter and is the major immunglobulin. IgA is secreted by B lymphocytes in the mucosa of the GI and respiratory tracts, and combines with inhaled or swallowed antigens so they are not absorbed into the body. IgE is the allergy antibody. IgD is attached to the cell membranes of B lymphocytes; it has some special functions that need not be considered now.

4. Hypersensitivity reactions are important and you should be familiar with them (see Table 5-1).
5. The IgE-mediated response triggers localized manifestations (allergy) or more serious systemic reactions to bee stings or penicillin reactions (anaphylaxis).
6. IgG-mediated hypersensitivity responses injure cells in two ways: by binding to cells and activating complement, which causes inflammation and tissue injury, or by forming antigen–antibody aggregates in tissues or in the circulation, which activates complement and induces inflammation.
7. A delayed hypersensitivity response (tuberculin-type hypersensitivity reaction) is a cell-mediated reaction and is not antibody related. Sensitized T lymphocytes accumulate at the site of contact with the foreign material and release lymphokines that attract macrophages and cytotoxic T lymphocytes. These attracted cells secrete cytokines (lymphokines and monokines) that cause the tissue injury and inflammation. A positive Mantoux test is an example of this type of reaction. Much of the tissue necrosis in tuberculosis is the result of a delayed hypersensitivity reaction to products of the tubercle bacillus.
8. Autoimmune disease occurs when the body develops an immune response to its own antigens (self-antigens), which damages the body's own cells and tissues. The nature of the autoimmune disease is determined by which organ or tissue is being attacked by the autoantibody.
9. Various mechanisms have been postulated to explain autoimmune disease (see Fig. 5-6). Defective regulation of the immune system by helper and suppressor lymphocytes is another mechanism of injury and one of the more important causes of autoimmune disease.
10. Table 5-2 provides examples of various autoimmune diseases, but the details of those diseases are not important now. Some examples will be illustrated in class.

Study Questions

The following questions are provided as a test for comprehension and as a study guide for use with the text chapters. Additional study material is located at http://health.jbpub.com/humandisease/, which contains useful eLearning tools such as an A&P review, animated flashcards, interactive online glossary, crossword puzzles, and Web links.

Key Terms

Define the following terms:

1. Acquired immunity _____

2. Cell-mediated immunity _____

3. Humoral immunity _____

4. Hypersensitivity _____

5. Active immunity _____

6. Passive immunity _____

7. Autoantibody _____

True/False

Tell whether the following statements are true or false as they apply to viral infections. If false, explain why the statement is incorrect.

1. Many viral infections cause acute cell necrosis and degeneration. _____

_____

2. Some viruses cause warts. _____

_____

3. Some viruses may persist indefinitely in the tissues of the host and become reactivated periodically, causing disease.

_____

4. Some viruses cause slowly progressive cell injury. _____

_____

5. Viruses are inhibited by adrenal corticosteroids. _____

_____

6. Some viruses respond to antiviral chemotherapeutic agents. _____

_____

Identify

1. Identify and describe the four major types of hypersensitivity reactions that cause tissue injury. (*Hint:* See Table 5-1.)

   a. _____

   b. _____

   c. _____

   d. _____

2. Identify and describe the four major categories of immunosuppressive agents used by physicians to treat autoimmune diseases or to perform organ transplants.

a. _____

b. _____

c. _____

d. _____

3. Identify and briefly describe three mechanisms postulated to explain the pathogenesis of autoimmune diseases.

a. _____

b. _____

c. _____

Discussion Questions

1. Describe the role of the lymphocyte in acquired immunity. (*Hint:* See Fig. 5-2.) _____

   _____

   _____

   _____

2. Describe the role of the macrophage in acquired immunity. _____

   _____

   _____

   _____

   _____

3. Describe the role of complement in immune responses. _____

   _____

   _____

   _____

4. Draw and label a simple diagram of an immunoglobulin molecule.

5. List the major types of immunoglobulin molecules and describe the function of each type. _____

   _____

   _____

   _____

6. What is the difference between immunity and hypersensitivity? _____

_____

_____

_____

7. What is the effect of autoantibody directed against the patient's own blood cells? _____

_____

_____

_____

8. Describe what happens in a cell-mediated immune response secondary to a pathogenic microorganism. _____

_____

_____

_____

9. Explain what happens when autoimmune diseases occur. How are they treated? _____

_____

_____

_____

10. Describe what happens when a pathogenic organism enters the body. _____

_____

_____

_____

11. Explain what happens when a person has a fungal infection. Are they treatable? _____

_____

_____

_____

BODY DEFENSES

INTACT BODY SURFACES AND ADAPTATIONS
  CILIA, MUCUS, ACID pH, ETC

ANTIBACTERIAL ENVIRONMENT AND SECRETIONS

THE INFLAMMATORY REACTION
  NON-SPECIFIC UNLEARNED REACTION
  TO INJURY

ACQUIRED IMMUNITY
  ANTIGEN PROCESSING: MONOCYTE
  ANTIGEN RESPONDING: LYMPHOCYTE

IMMUNITY CONCEPTS

ONE OF THE BODY'S DEFENSES

ANTIGEN = SUBSTANCE THAT INDUCES FORMATION
          OF ANTIBODY

ANTIBODY = SUBSTANCE FORMED IN RESPONSE
           TO ANTIGEN

LYMPHOCYTES RESPOND TO FOREIGN ANTIGEN

NORMALLY WE DON'T RESPOND TO OUR OWN
         ANTIGENS (SELF ANTIGENS)

ANTIGENIC SUBSTANCES

  BIG MOLECULES, USUALLY PROTEINS
   NOT THE WHOLE MOLECULE, ONLY PARTS
   OF THE MOLECULE (ANTIGENIC DETERMINANTS)

  SMALL MOLECULES (HAPTENS) THAT COMBINE
  WITH PROTEINS

THE TYPE OF IMMUNE RESPONSE IS DETERMINE
BY THE TYPE OF LYMPHOCYTE THAT RESPONDS
TO THE ANTIGEN

ORIGIN AND DIFFERENTIATION OF LYMPHOCYTES

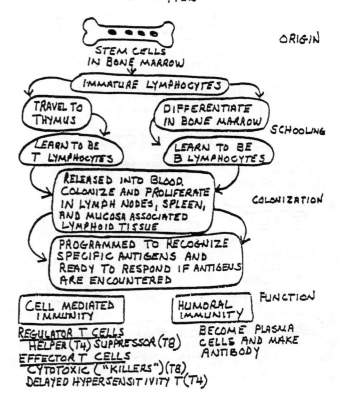

STEM CELLS IN BONE MARROW — ORIGIN

IMMATURE LYMPHOCYTES

TRAVEL TO THYMUS | DIFFERENTIATE IN BONE MARROW — SCHOOLING

LEARN TO BE T LYMPHOCYTES | LEARN TO BE B LYMPHOCYTES

RELEASED INTO BLOOD, COLONIZE AND PROLIFERATE IN LYMPH NODES, SPLEEN, AND MUCOSA ASSOCIATED LYMPHOID TISSUE — COLONIZATION

PROGRAMMED TO RECOGNIZE SPECIFIC ANTIGENS AND READY TO RESPOND IF ANTIGENS ARE ENCOUNTERED

CELL MEDIATED IMMUNITY | HUMORAL IMMUNITY — FUNCTION

REGULATOR T CELLS
  HELPER (T4) SUPPRESSOR (T8)
EFFECTOR T CELLS
  CYTOTOXIC ("KILLERS") (T8)
  DELAYED HYPERSENSITIVITY T (T4)

BECOME PLASMA CELLS AND MAKE ANTIBODY

IMMUNITY: RESPONSE TO FOREIGN ("NON-SELF") ANTIGEN

LYMPHOCYTES PRE-PROGRAMMED TO RESPOND.

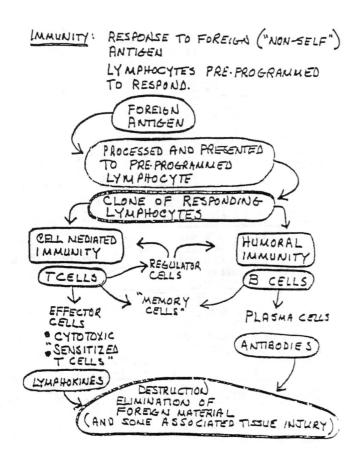

FOREIGN ANTIGEN

PROCESSED AND PRESENTED TO PRE-PROGRAMMED LYMPHOCYTE

CLONE OF RESPONDING LYMPHOCYTES

CELL MEDIATED IMMUNITY — REGULATOR CELLS — HUMORAL IMMUNITY

T CELLS — "MEMORY CELLS" — B CELLS

EFFECTOR CELLS
• CYTOTOXIC
• "SENSITIZED T CELLS"

PLASMA CELLS

LYMPHOKINES

ANTIBODIES

DESTRUCTION ELIMINATION OF FOREIGN MATERIAL (AND SOME ASSOCIATED TISSUE INJURY)

TYPES OF LYMPHOCYTES IN THE CIRCULATION

ABOUT 60% ARE T LYMPHOCYTES WITH VARIOUS FUNCTIONS

REGULATORS — T4 (CD4): HELPER T CELLS PROMOTE IMMUNE RESPONSE
T8 (CD8): SUPPRESSOR T CELLS INHIBIT IMMUNE RESPONSE

EFFECTORS — T8 (CD8): CYTOTOXIC T CELLS DESTROY FOREIGN, ABNORMAL, OR INFECTED CELLS

T4 (CD4): "SENSITIZED" T CELLS ATTRACT AND STIMULATE MACROPHAGES, CYTOTOXIC T CELLS, AND OTHER KILLER LYMPHOCYTES, WHICH DESTROY THE FOREIGN, ABNORMAL, OR INFECTED CELLS

ABOUT 30% ARE B LYMPHOCYTES
RESPOND TO FOREIGN ANTIGENS, BECOME PLASMA CELLS, AND PRODUCE ANTIBODIES

ABOUT 10% ARE NEITHER T NOR B CELLS
NATURAL KILLER CELLS (NK CELLS) CAN DESTROY ABNORMAL OR INFECTED CELLS EVEN WITHOUT PRIOR ANTIGENIC CONTACT

IG = ANTIBODIES = IMMUNOGLOBULINS

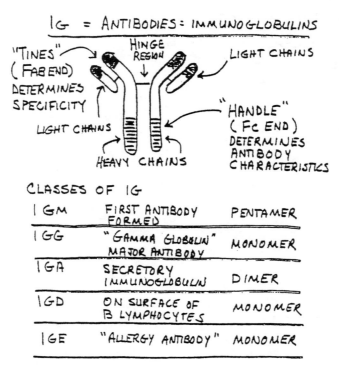

"TINES" (FAB END) DETERMINES SPECIFICITY

HINGE REGION

LIGHT CHAINS

LIGHT CHAINS

HEAVY CHAINS

"HANDLE" (Fc END) DETERMINES ANTIBODY CHARACTERISTICS

CLASSES OF IG

IGM	FIRST ANTIBODY FORMED	PENTAMER
IGG	"GAMMA GLOBULIN" MAJOR ANTIBODY	MONOMER
IGA	SECRETORY IMMUNOGLOBULIN	DIMER
IGD	ON SURFACE OF B LYMPHOCYTES	MONOMER
IGE	"ALLERGY ANTIBODY"	MONOMER

- LYMPHOCYTES ARE PROGRAMMED TO RECOGNIZE ANY ANTIGEN THEY WILL EVER ENCOUNTER.

- LYMPHOCYTES RESPOND TO PROCESSED ANTIGEN (PIECES OF ANTIGEN).

- T CELLS REGULATE IMMUNE RESPONSE (HELPER/SUPPRESSOR) AND ALSO "ATTACK" FOREIGN MATERIAL (CYTOTOXIC T CELLS) OR ATTRACT OTHER CELLS (MONOCYTES, CYTOTOXIC T CELLS, KILLER CELLS) WHICH DO THE DAMAGE [SENSITIZED T CELLS = DELAYED HYPERSENSITIVITY CELLS]

- B CELLS BECOME PLASMA CELLS THAT MAKE ANTIBODIES.

- IT TAKES TIME TO "CRANK UP" AN IMMUNE RESPONSE ON FIRST CONTACT, BUT LATER CONTACT GENERATES RAPID RESPONSE (VIA MEMORY CELLS).

SOME LYMPHOCYTES DON'T HAVE T OR B MARKERS. THESE ARE KILLER CELLS THAT CAN DESTROY WITHOUT PRIOR ANTIGENIC CONTACT.

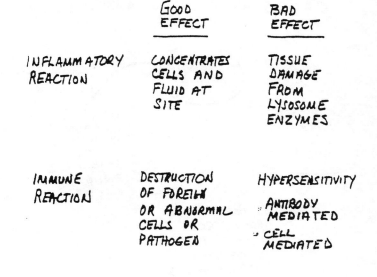

	GOOD EFFECT	BAD EFFECT
INFLAMMATORY REACTION	CONCENTRATES CELLS AND FLUID AT SITE	TISSUE DAMAGE FROM LYSOSOME ENZYMES
IMMUNE REACTION	DESTRUCTION OF FOREIGN OR ABNORMAL CELLS OR PATHOGEN	HYPERSENSITIVITY • ANTIBODY MEDIATED • CELL MEDIATED

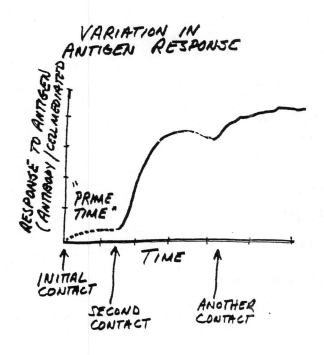

VARIATION IN ANTIGEN RESPONSE

RESPONSE TO ANTIGEN (ANTIBODY/CELL MEDIATED)

"PRIME TIME"

TIME

INITIAL CONTACT

SECOND CONTACT

ANOTHER CONTACT

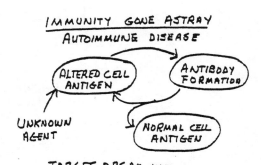

IMMUNITY GONE ASTRAY
AUTOIMMUNE DISEASE

ALTERED CELL ANTIGEN → ANTIBODY FORMATION

UNKNOWN AGENT

NORMAL CELL ANTIGEN

TARGET ORGAN INJURY
BLOOD CELLS = HEMOLYTIC ANEMIA
THYROID GLAND = DYSFUNCTION
CONNECTIVE TISSUE = "COLLAGEN DISEASE"

CROSS REACTING ANTIBODY

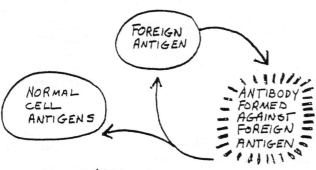

ANTIBODY
CROSS REACTS
WITH SIMILAR
ANTIGENIC
DETERMINANTS
ON NORMAL
CELLS AND TISSUES

MECHANISMS OF IMMUNOLOGIC INJURY

ANTIBODY MEDIATED

IMMEDIATE HYPERSENSITIVITY REACTION
IGE ANTIBODIES FIX TO MAST CELLS
LATER CONTACT WITH ANTIGEN TRIGGERS
MEDIATOR RELEASE
    LOCALIZED = ALLERGY
    SYSTEMIC = ANAPHYLAXIS

CYTOTOXIC REACTION
OTHER ANTIBODIES (IGG, IGM) BIND
TO FIXED ANTIGEN ON CELLS
OR TISSUES

} ACTIVATED
COMPLEMENT
CAUSES
INFLAMMATION

IMMUNE COMPLEX REACTION
OTHER ANTIBODIES (IGG, IGM) BIND
TO CIRCULATING ANTIGENS AND
FORM COMPLEXES WHICH DEPOSIT
IN TISSUES

MEDIATED BY SENSITIZED T CELLS
DELAYED HYPERSENSITIVITY REACTION
SENSITIZED T CELLS ACCUMULATE, ATTRACT
AND ACTIVATE MACROPHAGES, CYTOTOXIC
T CELLS = INFLAMMATION, NECROSIS

POORLY CONTROLLED IMMUNE RESPONSE

INCREASE

DECREASE

HELPER T CELLS
↓
IMMUNE RESPONSE
↑
SUPPRESSOR T CELLS

AGENT STIMULATES
IMMUNE SYSTEM
? VIRUS

POORLY CONTROLLED IMMUNE
RESPONSE
(GENETIC)

EXCESSIVE HELPER T ACTIVITY

EXCESSIVE B CELL
STIMULATION

HYPERACTIVE B LYMPHOCYTES
↓
ACTIVATION OF PREVIOUSLY SUPPRESSED
LYMPHOCYTES DIRECTED AGAINST SELF ANTIGENS
↓
AUTOANTIBODIES

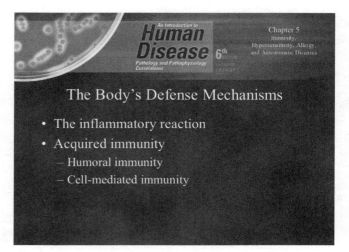

The Body's Defense Mechanisms

- The inflammatory reaction
- Acquired immunity
  - Humoral immunity
  - Cell-mediated immunity

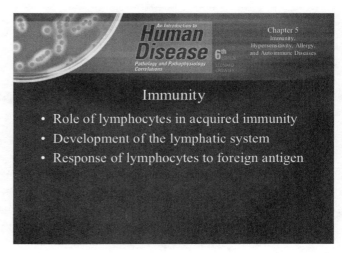

Immunity

- Role of lymphocytes in acquired immunity
- Development of the lymphatic system
- Response of lymphocytes to foreign antigen

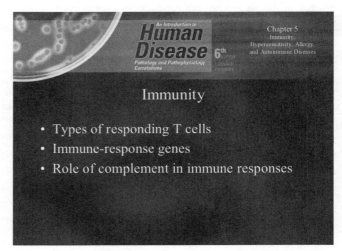

Immunity

- Types of responding T cells
- Immune-response genes
- Role of complement in immune responses

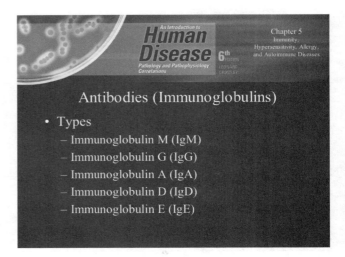

Antibodies (Immunoglobulins)

- Types
  - Immunoglobulin M (IgM)
  - Immunoglobulin G (IgG)
  - Immunoglobulin A (IgA)
  - Immunoglobulin D (IgD)
  - Immunoglobulin E (IgE)

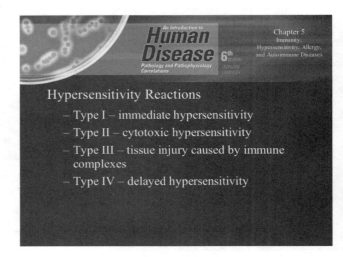

Hypersensitivity Reactions

- Type I – immediate hypersensitivity
- Type II – cytotoxic hypersensitivity
- Type III – tissue injury caused by immune complexes
- Type IV – delayed hypersensitivity

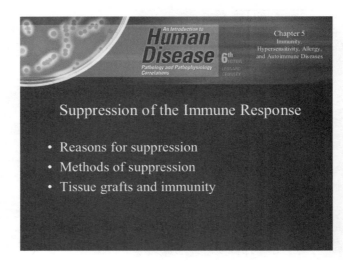

Suppression of the Immune Response

- Reasons for suppression
- Methods of suppression
- Tissue grafts and immunity

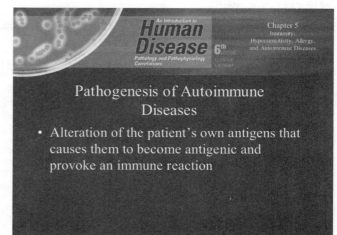

Pathogenesis of Autoimmune Diseases

- Alteration of the patient's own antigens that causes them to become antigenic and provoke an immune reaction

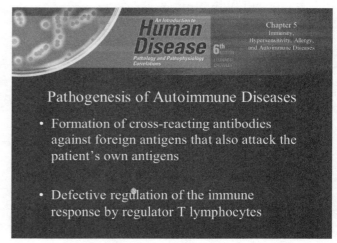

Pathogenesis of Autoimmune Diseases

- Formation of cross-reacting antibodies against foreign antigens that also attack the patient's own antigens

- Defective regulation of the immune response by regulator T lymphocytes

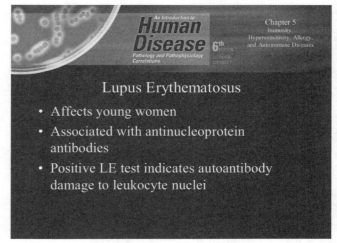

Lupus Erythematosus

- Affects young women
- Associated with antinucleoprotein antibodies
- Positive LE test indicates autoantibody damage to leukocyte nuclei

Chapter Outline

The chapter outline provides you with an organizational guide to the topics and ideas presented in this chapter of the text.

Types of Harmful Microorganisms
Bacteria
    Classification of Bacteria
    Identification of Bacteria
    Major Classes of Pathogenic Bacteria
    Antibiotic Treatment of Bacterial Infections
    Antibiotic Sensitivity Tests
    Adverse Effects of Antibiotics
Chlamydiae
Rickettsiae
Mycoplasmas
Viruses
    Classification of Viruses
    Mode of Action
    Bodily Defenses Against Viral Infections
    Treatment with Antiviral Agents
Fungi
    Superficial Fungal Infections
    Highly Pathogenic Fungi
    Other Fungi of Medical Importance
    Treatment of Systemic Fungal Infections

Study Questions

The following questions are provided as a test for comprehension and as a study guide for use with the text chapters. Additional study material is located at http://health.jbpub.com/humandisease/, which contains useful eLearning tools such as an A&P review, animated flashcards, interactive online glossary, crossword puzzles, and Web links.

Key Terms

Define the following terms:

1. Virus _____

2. Human papillomavirus _____

3. *Histoplasma capsulatum* _____

4. *Neisseria* _____

5. Latent virus infection _____

6. Hemolysis _____

7. Antigens _____

8. Pathogenic _____

True/False

1. Tell whether each statement is true or false as it applies to streptococci. If false, explain why the statement is incorrect.

   a. The organisms are classified based on the carbohydrate antigens present in their cell walls and on the type of hemolysis produced by the organism growing on a blood agar plate. _____

   _____

   b. Most alpha hemolytic streptococci are very pathogenic. _____

   _____

   c. Group A beta streptococci may cause serious respiratory tract infections such as streptococcal pharyngitis, and such infections may be followed by rheumatic fever. _____

   _____

   d. Group B beta streptococci may colonize the genital tract of pregnant women, and may lead to an infection in the infant caused by the streptococcus acquired by the infant during delivery. _____

   _____

2. Tell whether each statement is true or false as it applies to the organism causing anthrax (*Bacillus anthracis*). If false, explain why the statement is incorrect.

   a. The organism is a gram-positive, spore-forming aerobic bacillus. _____

   _____

   b. The organism can be used as a bioterrorism–germ warfare agent. _____

   _____

c. Inhalation of anthrax spores may cause a severe pulmonary infection. _____

_____

d. Pulmonary anthrax caused by inhalation of anthrax spores can be prevented by a short (one- to two-week) course of antibiotics, because the organism is sensitive to antibiotics. _____

_____

Identify

1. Identify and briefly describe the four potentially harmful side effects of antibiotics.

   a. _____

   b. _____

   c. _____

   d. _____

2. Identify the important diseases caused by:

   a. Pneumococci _____

   b. Gonococci _____

   c. Acid-fast bacteria _____

3. Identify two highly pathogenic fungi and the type of diseases they produce.

   a. _____

   b. _____

4. Identify five possible effects of a virus invasion of a susceptible cell. (*Hint:* See Fig. 6-4.)

   a. _____

   b. _____

   c. _____

   d. _____

   e. _____

5. List the four major factors used to classify bacteria.

   a. _____

   b. _____

   c. _____

   d. _____

Matching

Match the diseases in the right column with the responsible organisms in the left column.

1. _____ Group A beta streptococcus
2. _____ Group B beta streptococcus
3. _____ Hemolytic staphylococcus
4. _____ Human papillomavirus
5. _____ *Histoplasma capsulatum*
6. _____ Herpes virus
7. _____ Varicella zoster virus
8. _____ Mumps virus
9. _____ *Bacillus anthracis*
10. _____ Meningococcus (*Neisseria meningiditis*)

A. Severe throat infection
B. Warts
C. Infection of newborn infant
D. "Fever blisters"
E. Pulmonary infection
F. Germ warfare agent
G. Wound infection
H. Skin rash
I. Parotid gland infection
J. Meningitis

Discussion Questions

1. How is the gram stain used to classify bacteria? _____

2. How do antibiotics inhibit the growth of bacteria? (See Fig. 6-2.) _____

3. How does penicillin kill bacteria? _____

4. How do bacteria become resistant to an antibiotic? _____

5. What factors render a patient susceptible to an infection by a fungus of low pathogenicity? _____

PATHOGENIC
MICROORGANISMS

BACTERIA
  CHLAMYDIAE
  RICKETTSIAE
  MYCOPLASMAS

FUNGI
  YEASTS
  MOLDS

VIRUSES
  DNA
  RNA

ANIMAL PARASITES

CLASSIFICATION OF BACTERIA
  SHAPE
  GRAM STAIN
  CULTURAL CHARACTERISTICS
  ANTIGENIC STRUCTURE

IMPORTANT PATHOGENS

COCCI

GRAM POS.	GRAM NEG.
STAPHYLOCOCCI	GONOCOCCI
STREPTOCOCCI	MENINGOCOCCI
PNEUMOCOCCI	

BACILLI

CORYNEBACTERIA   ENTERIC BACTERIA
(AEROBIC)
LISTERIA
CLOSTRIDIA
(ANAEROBIC)

SPIRALS

TREPONEMA PALLIDUM
BORRELIA BURGDORFERI

ACID FAST

TUBERCLE BACILLUS
LEPROSY BACILLUS
MYCOBACTERIA OTHER THAN TUBERCLE
    BACILLUS (MOTT)

TREATMENT

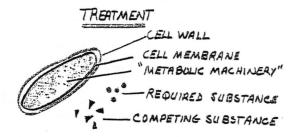

    CELL WALL
    CELL MEMBRANE
    "METABOLIC MACHINERY"
    REQUIRED SUBSTANCE
    COMPETING SUBSTANCE

HOW ANTIBIOTICS WORK

1. PREVENT CELL WALL SYNTHESIS
2. DAMAGE CELL MEMBRANE
3. DISRUPT METABOLIC MACHINERY
4. CONFUSE MICROORGANISM WITH
   "LOOK ALIKE" COMPOUND

HAZARDS OF ANTIBIOTICS
(RISK VS. BENEFIT)
    TOXICITY
    HYPERSENSITIVITY
    ALTER BACTERIAL FLORA
    FAVOR GROWTH OF RESISTANT "BUGS"

RESISTANCE MECHANISMS

- CHANGE CELL WALL STRUCTURE
  (PERMEABILITY) SO ANTIBIOTIC CAN'T
  GET INTO BACTERIUM.
- ENZYMES INACTIVATE ANTIBIOTIC
- EJECT ANTIBIOTIC BEFORE IT CAN HARM
  BACTERIUM
- CHANGE STRUCTURE OF CELL COMPONENT
  (TARGET) ATTACKED BY ANTIBIOTIC SO
  ANTIBIOTIC CAN'T BIND TO TARGET
  (RIBOSOMES, BACTERIAL ENZYMES
  FORMING CELL WALL, ETC.)

PRINCIPLES OF TREATMENT

- IS ANTIBIOTIC NEEDED?
- WHICH ANTIBIOTIC IS LIKELY TO BE
  MOST EFFECTIVE AND LEAST TOXIC
  (AND LEAST EXPENSIVE)
- CONFIRM WITH SENSITIVITY TEST
  WHERE APPROPRIATE
- GIVE ENOUGH ANTIBIOTIC LONG ENOUGH.

FUNGI

OPPORTUNIST
PATHOGENS
   YEAST INFECTION

HIGHLY PATHOGENIC

HISTOPLASMOSIS
COCCIDIODOMYCOSIS

VIRUSES

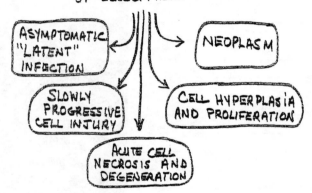

VIRUS INVASION
OF SUSCEPTIBLE CELL

ASYMPTOMATIC "LATENT" INFECTION

NEOPLASM

SLOWLY PROGRESSIVE CELL INJURY

CELL HYPERPLASIA AND PROLIFERATION

ACUTE CELL NECROSIS AND DEGENERATION

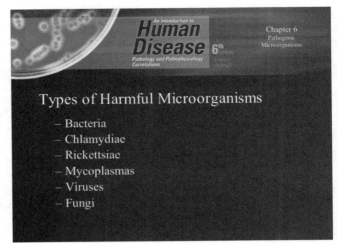

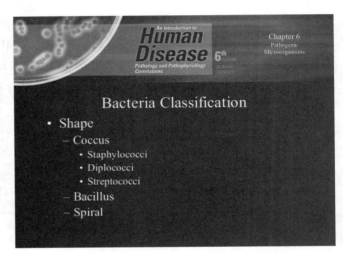

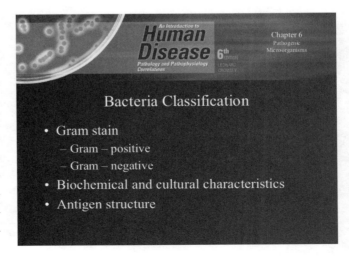

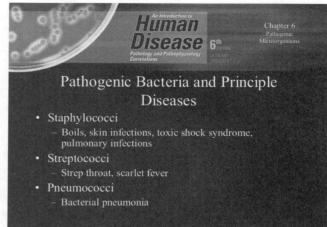

Pathogenic Bacteria and Principle Diseases

- Staphylococci
  - Boils, skin infections, toxic shock syndrome, pulmonary infections
- Streptococci
  - Strep throat, scarlet fever
- Pneumococci
  - Bacterial pneumonia

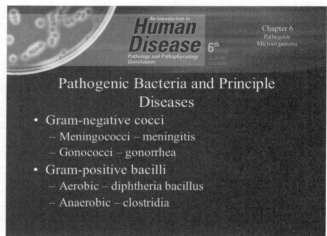

Pathogenic Bacteria and Principle Diseases

- Gram-negative cocci
  - Meningococci – meningitis
  - Gonococci – gonorrhea
- Gram-positive bacilli
  - Aerobic – diphtheria bacillus
  - Anaerobic – clostridia

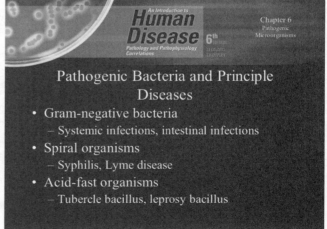

Pathogenic Bacteria and Principle Diseases

- Gram-negative bacteria
  - Systemic infections, intestinal infections
- Spiral organisms
  - Syphilis, Lyme disease
- Acid-fast organisms
  - Tubercle bacillus, leprosy bacillus

Notes

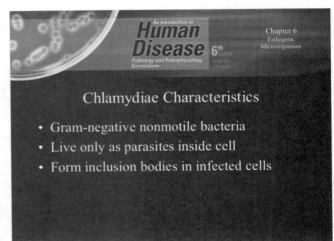

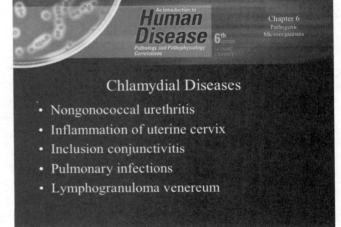

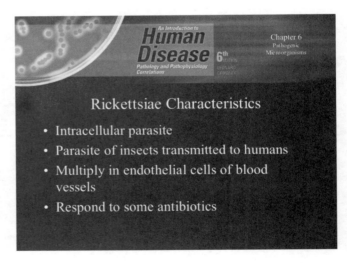

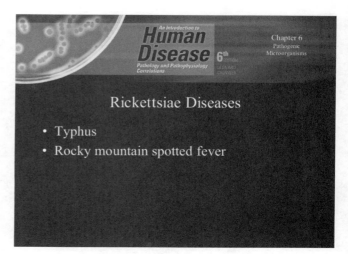

Rickettsiae Diseases

- Typhus
- Rocky mountain spotted fever

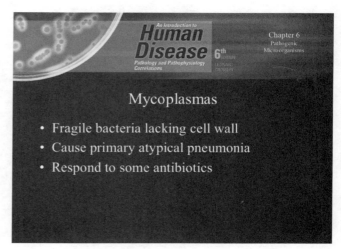

Mycoplasmas

- Fragile bacteria lacking cell wall
- Cause primary atypical pneumonia
- Respond to some antibiotics

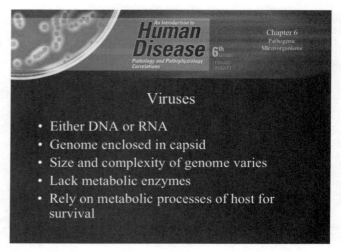

Viruses

- Either DNA or RNA
- Genome enclosed in capsid
- Size and complexity of genome varies
- Lack metabolic enzymes
- Rely on metabolic processes of host for survival

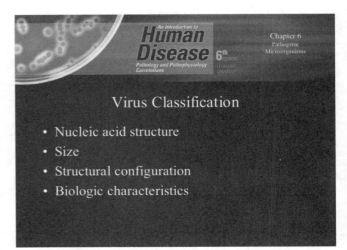

Chapter 6
Pathogenic Microorganisms

Virus Classification

- Nucleic acid structure
- Size
- Structural configuration
- Biologic characteristics

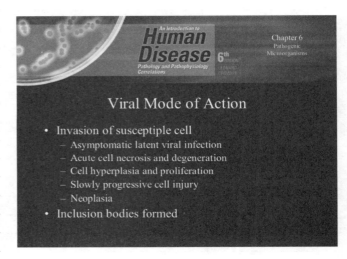

Chapter 6
Pathogenic Microorganisms

Viral Mode of Action

- Invasion of susceptible cell
  - Asymptomatic latent viral infection
  - Acute cell necrosis and degeneration
  - Cell hyperplasia and proliferation
  - Slowly progressive cell injury
  - Neoplasia
- Inclusion bodies formed

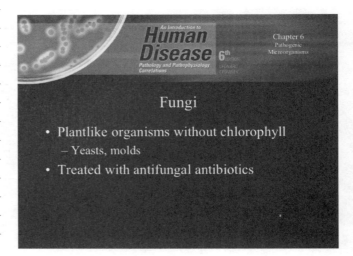

Chapter 6
Pathogenic Microorganisms

Fungi

- Plantlike organisms without chlorophyll
  - Yeasts, molds
- Treated with antifungal antibiotics

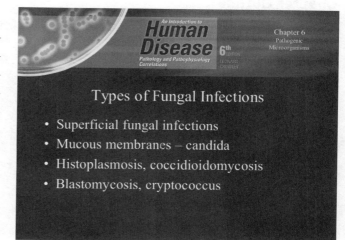

Types of Fungal Infections

- Superficial fungal infections
- Mucous membranes – candida
- Histoplasmosis, coccidioidomycosis
- Blastomycosis, cryptococcus

Chapter Outline

The chapter outline provides you with an organizational guide to the topics and ideas presented in this chapter of the text.

The Parasite and Its Host
Protozoal Infestations
    Malaria
    Amebiasis
    Genital Tract Infections Caused by Trichomonads
    Giardiasis
    Toxoplasmosis
    Cryptosporidiosis
Metazoal Infestations
    Roundworms
    Tapeworms
    Flukes
Arthropods

Study Questions

The following questions are provided as a test for comprehension and as a study guide for use with the text chapters. Additional study material is located at http://health.jbpub.com/humandisease/, which contains useful eLearning tools such as an A&P review, animated flashcards, interactive online glossary, crossword puzzles, and Web links.

Key Terms

Define the following terms:

1. Protozoa _____

2. Metazoa _____

3. *Toxoplasma gondii* _____

4. *Pneumocystis carinii* _____

Fill-in-the-Blank

1. _____ is the large roundworm that lives in the intestinal tract of humans and that is acquired from ingestion of worm eggs.

2. _____ is the small (1 cm long) roundworm that inhabits the colon of infected children and periodically migrates out of the anus at night to deposit eggs on the perianal skin.

3. _____ is the small roundworm that forms cysts in the muscles of infected animals, and may cause a serious systemic illness in persons who ingest the cysts contained in incompletely cooked meat.

4. _____ is the long ribbon-like worm that lives in the intestinal tract, which is acquired by eating the flesh of infected animals or fish.

5. _____ is the fluke infestation that causes an itchy skin rash, as a result of swimming in a lake containing the infectious form of the parasite.

6. _____ is the sexually transmitted parasite that causes an intense itching of the pubic skin.

7. _____ is a parasite that infests many birds and animals, which can be transmitted to humans by ingestion of incompletely cooked meat (such as hamburgers) or by contact with infected cats that excrete and infectious form of the parasite in their feces.

Identify

1. Indicate the name of the parasite that causes the following diseases or conditions:

    a. A protozoal disease transmitted by mosquitoes _____

    b. An intestinal infestation caused by a pathogenic amoeba _____
    _____

    c. A sexually transmitted infection caused by a small motile parasite that does not form cysts _____
    _____

    d. An intestinal infection caused by a small pear-shaped parasite that causes intestinal cramps and diarrhea
    _____

e. A parasitic infection that may be transmitted from a recently infected pregnant woman to her fetus _____

f. A parasitic infection that may be acquired by contact with cats _____

g. A small parasite that forms highly resistant cysts that may contaminate municipal water supplies, lakes and rivers, and swimming pools; ingestion of the cysts causes cramps and diarrhea _____

h. A small parasite that causes a skin rash _____

2. Identify the three large groups of metazoal parasites.

a. _____

b. _____

c. _____

Matching

Match the parasite in the right column with the clinical manifestation or condition in the left column. Some letters may be used more than once, and some may not be used:

1. ____ "Swimmer's itch"

2. ____ Profuse vaginal discharge

3. ____ Injures the fetus of a pregnant woman

4. ____ Severe life-threatening diarrhea in an immunocompromised person

5. ____ Fever, cough, and pulmonary inflammation

6. ____ Diarrhea from swimming in chlorinated swimming pool

7. ____ Chills and fever

8. ____ Perianal itching awakening a child at night

9. ____ Itching of pubic skin

10. ____ Severe pulmonary infection in an immunocompromised person

A. Pinworms

B. *Plasmodium* species

C. Crab louse

D. Ascaris larvae

E. *Trichomonas*

F. *Cryptosporidium*

G. Tapeworm

H. *Toxoplasma*

I. *Schistosomes*

J. *Pneumocystis*

ANIMAL PARASITES

CLASSIFICATION (SEE ANIMAL PARASITES HANDOUT CHAPTER)

PROTOZOA: SINGLE CELLS
- MALARIA (PLASMODIUM)
- ENTAMOEBA HISTOLYTICA
- TRICHOMONAS
- GIARDIA
- TOXOPLASMA   CRYPTOSPORIDIA
- PNEUMOCYSTIS

METAZOA: MULTICELLED
- ROUNDWORMS
- TAPEWORMS
- FLUKES

ARTHROPODS: INSECTS
- SCABIES
- LICE

MALARIA

INFECTED HUMAN → MOSQUITO → HUMAN INFECTED: PARASITES DEVELOP IN LIVER INITIALLY

→ PARASITES ATTACK AND MULTIPLY IN RED CELL. FORM HEMOGLOBIN BREAKDOWN PIGMENTS

→ RED CELLS RUPTURE. NEW PARASITES RELEASED MALARIAL PIGMENT RELEASED (CHILLS AND FEVER)

TOXOPLASMOSIS:

INTRACELLULAR PARASITE OF BIRDS, ANIMALS AND PEOPLE (50% HAVE ANTIBODIES FROM PRIOR INFECTION)

→ CATS INFECTED FROM EATING INFECTED MICE OR OTHER MEAT, AND EXCRETE INFECTIOUS FORM OF PARASITE

→ PEOPLE INFECTED FROM INCOMPLETELY COOKED MEAT OR CONTACT WITH CATS.

- ACUTE INFECTION (LIKE INFECTIOUS MONONUCLEOSIS)
- ASYMPTOMATIC INFECTION
- TRANSMISSION TO FETUS

PREVENT INFECTION OF SUSCEPTIBLE PREGNANT WOMAN

TRICHOMONADS: VAGINAL INFECTION SEXUALLY TRANSMITTED TREAT BOTH PARTNERS. (NO CYST FORMS)

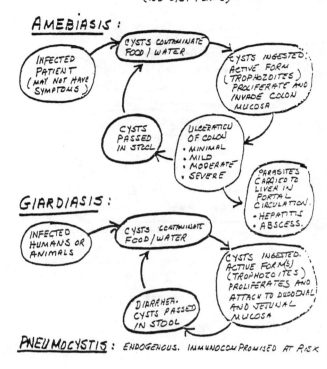

AMEBIASIS:

INFECTED PATIENT (MAY NOT HAVE SYMPTOMS) → CYSTS CONTAMINATE FOOD/WATER → CYSTS INGESTED: ACTIVE FORM (TROPHOZOITES) PROLIFERATE AND INVADE COLON MUCOSA

→ ULCERATION OF COLON
- MINIMAL
- MILD
- MODERATE
- SEVERE

→ CYSTS PASSED IN STOOL

→ PARASITES CARRIED TO LIVER IN PORTAL CIRCULATION.
- HEPATITIS
- ABSCESS.

GIARDIASIS:

INFECTED HUMANS OR ANIMALS → CYSTS CONTAMINATE FOOD/WATER → CYSTS INGESTED. ACTIVE FORM(S) (TROPHOZOITES) PROLIFERATES AND ATTACH TO DUODENAL AND JEJUNAL MUCOSA

→ DIARRHEA. CYSTS PASSED IN STOOL

PNEUMOCYSTIS: ENDOGENOUS. IMMUNOCOMPROMISED AT RISK

CRYPTOSPORIDIOSIS

- FARM ANIMALS INFECTED. EXCRETE C. PARVUM OOCYSTS

- SURFACE WATER CONTAMINATED

- PEOPLE INFECTED FROM INGESTING OOCYSTS
  - UNFILTERED WATER SUPPLIES
  - SWIMMING POOLS
  - WAVE POOLS

- ACUTE DIARRHEA
  - SELF LIMITED IN IMMUNOCOMPETENT
  - CHRONIC SEVERE IN IMMUNOCOMPROMISED

NO SPECIFIC TREATMENT

FLAT WORMS

TAPEWORMS: (PORK, BEEF, FISH)

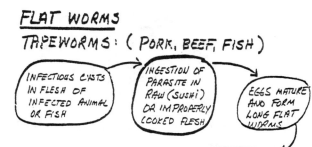

- INFECTIOUS CYSTS IN FLESH OF INFECTED ANIMAL OR FISH
- INGESTION OF PARASITE IN RAW (SUSHI) OR IMPROPERLY COOKED FLESH
- EGGS MATURE AND FORM LONG FLAT WORMS
- WORMS EAT OUR FOOD AND DON'T DO ANYTHING FOR US

FLUKES

SHORT FLESHY FLAT WORMS WITH SUCKERS
COMPLEX LIFE CYCLE WITH INTERMEDIATE HOSTS
CLASSIFIED ON LOCATION OF FLUKE IN INFECTED
PERSON:
- INTESTINAL FLUKES
- LUNG FLUKES
- LIVER FLUKES

NOT A PROBLEM IN THIS COUNTRY

ARTHROPODS: TRANSMITTED BY CLOSE CONTACT.

SCABIES: SMALL PARASITE. BURROWS IN SKIN. INTENSE ITCHING

LICE:
- HEAD LOUSE
- BODY LOUSE
- "CRABS" (PUBIC LOUSE)

WORMS:

ROUND WORMS

ASCARIS: EARTHWORM SIZE

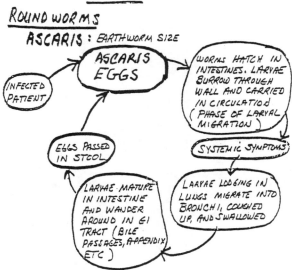

- INFECTED PATIENT
- ASCARIS EGGS
- WORMS HATCH IN INTESTINES. LARVAE BURROW THROUGH WALL AND CARRIED IN CIRCULATION (PHASE OF LARVAL MIGRATION)
- SYSTEMIC SYMPTOMS
- LARVAE LODGING IN LUNGS MIGRATE INTO BRONCHI, COUGHED UP, AND SWALLOWED
- LARVAE MATURE IN INTESTINE AND WANDER AROUND IN GI TRACT (BILE PASSAGES, APPENDIX, ETC)
- EGGS PASSED IN STOOL

PINWORMS: PIN SIZED (~1cm.)

A NUISANCE WORM. PERSON TO PERSON TRANSMISSION!

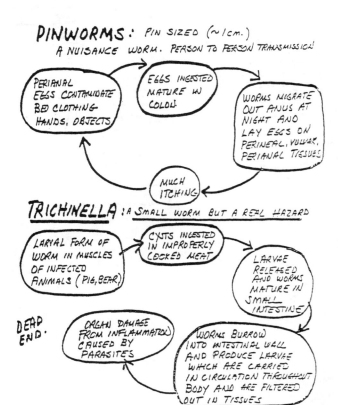

- PERIANAL EGGS CONTAMINATE BED CLOTHING, HANDS, OBJECTS
- EGGS INGESTED MATURE IN COLON
- WORMS MIGRATE OUT ANUS AT NIGHT AND LAY EGGS ON PERINEAL, VULVAR, PERIANAL TISSUES
- MUCH ITCHING

TRICHINELLA: A SMALL WORM BUT A REAL HAZARD

- LARVAL FORM OF WORM IN MUSCLES OF INFECTED ANIMALS (PIG, BEAR)
- CYSTS INGESTED IN IMPROPERLY COOKED MEAT
- LARVAE RELEASED AND WORMS MATURE IN SMALL INTESTINE
- WORMS BURROW INTO INTESTINAL WALL AND PRODUCE LARVAE WHICH ARE CARRIED IN CIRCULATION THROUGHOUT BODY AND ARE FILTERED OUT IN TISSUES
- ORGAN DAMAGE FROM INFLAMMATION CAUSED BY PARASITES

DEAD END.

Notes

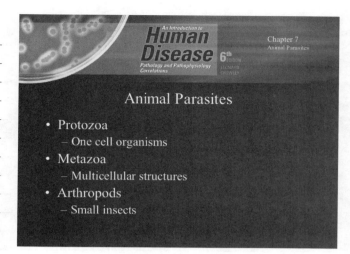

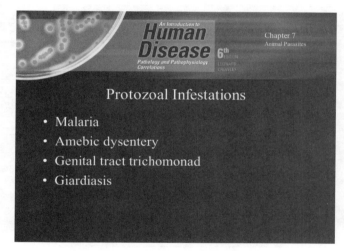

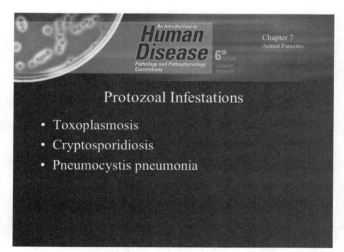

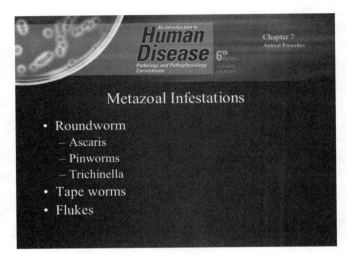

Metazoal Infestations

- Roundworm
  - Ascaris
  - Pinworms
  - Trichinella
- Tape worms
- Flukes

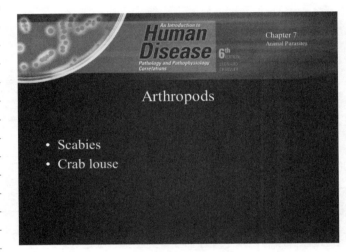

Arthropods

- Scabies
- Crab louse

Chapter 8   Communicable Diseases

Chapter Outline

The chapter outline provides you with an organizational guide to the topics and ideas presented in this chapter of the text.

Methods of Transmission and Control
Methods of Transmission
Methods of Control
    Immunization
    Identification, Isolation, and Treatment of Infected Persons
    Control of Means of Indirect Transmission
    Requirements for Effective Control
Sexually Transmitted Diseases
    Syphilis
    Gonorrhea
    Herpes
    Genital Chlamydial Infections
Human Immunodeficiency Virus Infections and AIDS
    HIV and Its Target
    Early Manifestations of HIV Infection
    Late Manifestations of HIV Infection
    Measurements of Viral RNA and CD4 Lymphocytes as an Index of Disease Progression
    Complications of AIDS
    Prevalence of HIV Infection and AIDS in High-Risk Groups
    Prevention and Control of HIV Infection
    Treatment of HIV Infection

Study Questions

The following questions are provided as a test for comprehension and as a study guide for use with the text chapters. Additional study material is located at http://health.jbpub.com/humandisease/, which contains useful eLearning tools such as an A&P review, animated flashcards, interactive online glossary, crossword puzzles, and Web links.

Key Terms

Define the following terms:

1. Communicable disease _____

2. Chlamydia _____

3. HIV _____

4. AIDS _____

5. Opportunistic infections _____

True/False

Tell whether each statement is true or false. If false, explain why the statement is incorrect.

1. Currently, about 18 percent of all AIDS cases occur in women. _____

   _____

2. Among young persons ages 13 to 19, most HIV infections occur in males. _____

   _____

3. The drug zidovudine (ZDV), when given to a pregnant HIV-infected mother, significantly reduces the risk of mother-to-infant HIV transmission. _____

   _____

4. A newborn infant born to an HIV-infected mother is also treated with ZDV for several weeks after delivery. _____

   _____

5. A newborn infant born to an HIV-infected mother may be breastfed because the virus cannot be transmitted by breast milk.

   _____

6. Delivery of an HIV-infected mother by cesarean section reduces the risk of mother-to-infant HIV transmission.

   _____

Identify

1. Identify the four major sexually transmitted diseases. Indicate in tabular form the major clinical manifestations of each disease and method of treatment.

Disease	Manifestation	Treatment
a.		
b.		
c.		
d.		

2. Identify the three major classes of drugs used to treat HIV infection. Indicate briefly how each class acts to interrupt the replication of HIV.

a. _____

b. _____

c. _____

Discussion Questions

1. Describe how communicable diseases are transmitted. _____
_____
_____
_____

2. Describe how communicable diseases are controlled._____
_____
_____
_____

3. A woman has been infected with the genital herpes virus (type 2). Describe how she can reduce the risk of transmission of the infection to her sexual partner. _____
_____
_____
_____

4. An HIV-infected woman wishes to become pregnant. What steps can she take to minimize the risk of transmitting the infection to her infant when she becomes pregnant? _____
_____
_____
_____

5. A woman had a test performed for a chlamydial infection, and the test was positive. She is concerned about the consequences of the infection. What would you tell her about the consequences of the infection, the risk of infecting her partner, and steps she should take to eradicate the infection? _____
_____
_____
_____

6. Can an HIV infection be treated? Can it be cured? _____
_____
_____
_____

7. What should an HIV-infected person do to slow the progression of the infection and to prevent transmission of the infection to other persons? _____

_____

_____

8. An HIV-positive woman is considering becoming pregnant. What factors should she consider when she makes a decision as to whether to undertake a pregnancy? _____

_____

_____

9. What are the initial and late manifestations of HIV infection? _____

_____

_____

10. What groups are at high risk of HIV infection? _____

_____

_____

11. How can HIV transmission be reduced or prevented? _____

_____

_____

12. Explain whether each of the following descriptors applies to AIDS. Why or why not?

   a. Occurs frequently in female homosexuals _____

   _____

   b. Occurs frequently in male homosexuals _____

   _____

   c. Often fatal as a result of opportunistic infections _____

   _____

   d. Caused by a virus that damages the immune system _____

   _____

   e. May be contracted by blood transfusions _____

   _____

f. Usually responds to corticosteroids, which stimulate the immune system _____

_____

13. Explain whether each of the following descriptors applies to herpes infection of the genital tract. Why or why not?
   a. A sexually transmitted disease _____

   _____

   b. Initial attack confers permanent immunity _____

   _____

   c. May predispose to cervical carcinoma _____

   _____

   d. Patient may transmit herpes infection from oral cavity to genital tract by auto-inoculation _____

   _____

   e. Infected woman may transmit virus to her infant during childbirth _____

   _____

   f. Cannot be transmitted to sexual partner unless active lesions present in the genital tract _____

   _____

SEXUALLY TRANSMITTED DISEASES

HERPES

SUPERFICIAL PAINFUL
ULCERS AT SITE
NODES TENDER
SYSTEMIC SYMPTOMS

↓

REMISSION BUT VIRUS
"HIDES OUT" IN NERVE
TISSUE

↓

PERIODIC VIRUS
SHEDDING AND/OR
REACTIVATION

SYPHILIS

HARD NOT VERY
TENDER ULCER AT
SITE (CHANCRE)

↓

SKIN RASH
ENLARGED NODES
SYSTEMIC SYMPTOMS

↓

LATE DESTRUCTIVE
LESIONS CNS
CARDIOVASCULAR

TREATMENT

HERPES : CONTROL BUT NO CURE
SYPHILIS : ANTIBIOTICS

SEXUALLY TRANSMITTED DISEASES

CHLAMYDIA (SMALL "DEFECTIVE" INTRACELLULAR GRAM NEG. ROD)		GONORRHEA (GRAM NEG. DIPLOCOCCUS)
URETHRA CERVIX	SITE OF INFECTION	URETHRA CERVIX THROAT RECTUM
UPPER GENITAL TRACT	SPREAD COMPLICATIONS	UPPER GENITAL TRACT
DETECT CHLAMYDIAL ANTIGENS IN INFECTED CELLS	DIAGNOSIS	CULTURE
ANTIBIOTICS	TREATMENT	ANTIBIOTICS

COMMUNICABLE DISEASE

ENDEMIC
EPIDEMIC

PREREQUISITES

1. ENTRY OF ORGANISM
2. MULTIPLICATION OF ORGANISM
3. EXCRETION OF ORGANISM

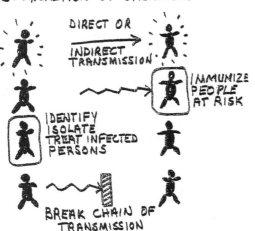

DIRECT OR
INDIRECT
TRANSMISSION

IMMUNIZE PEOPLE AT RISK

IDENTIFY
ISOLATE
TREAT INFECTED
PERSONS

BREAK CHAIN OF
TRANSMISSION

HIV INFECTION : RNA RETROVIRUS

EVENT	CONSEQUENCE
HIV INVADES CELL BECOMES PART OF CELL DNA	INFECTED FOR LIFE
VIRUS MULTIPLICATION AND SHEDDING	VIRUS IN BLOOD AND BODY FLUIDS
BODY FORM HIV ANTIBODY	INDICATION OF INFECTION. NOT PROTECTIVE
PROGRESSIVE DESTRUCTION OF HELPER T CELLS	COMPROMISED CELL MEDIATED IMMUNITY
IMMUNE DEFENSES COLLAPSE INFECTIONS TUMORS	AIDS

VIRAL RNA →REVERSE TRANSCRIPTASE→ DNA →HIV INTEGRASE→ VIRAL DNA INSERTED INTO NUCLEUS
ENTERS CELL

COMPLETE VIRUS BUDS FROM CELL ← PROTEIN CUT INTO SEGMENTS ←HIV PROTEASE← VIRAL RNA AND PROTEIN PRODUCED IN INFECTED CELL
VIRUS ASSEMBLED

TREATMENT

NON-NUCLEOSIDE REVERSE TRANSCRIPTASE INHIBITORS	BLOCK REVERSE TRANSCRIPTASE
NUCLEOSIDE REVERSE TRANSCRIPTASE INHIBITORS	SUBSTITUTE "LOOK ALIKE" COMPOUND (NUCLEOSIDE ANALOG)
PROTEASE INHIBITORS	BLOCK ENZYME THAT CUTS-ASSEMBLES PROTEIN AROUND VIRUS

WHEN TO TREAT

EARLY
- SUPPRESS VIRUS
- DELAYS IMMUNE SYSTEM DAMAGE AND COMPLICATIONS

LATE
- WAIT FOR IMMUNE SYSTEM DAMAGE
- AVOID DRUG TOXICITY
- REDUCE RISK OF DRUG RESISTANT STRAINS OF VIRUS

HOW DID VIRUS GET HERE

WHAT ARE THE HIGH RISK GROUPS ("THE 4 H GROUPS")

PRIMARY

HOMOSEXUALS (MALE)

HEMOPHILIACS

HAITIANS

HEROIN (DRUG) ABUSERS

SECONDARY

PROSTITUTES (SEX INDUSTRY WORKERS)

SEX PARTNERS OF INFECTED PERSONS

NEWBORN INFANTS OF INFECTED MOTHERS

PREVENTION

DISCRETION
"SAFE SEX"

PERSONS MUST ASSUME RESPONSIBILITY FOR THEIR OWN BEHAVIOR

AIDS UPDATE

DRUGS

"LOOK ALIKES" (NUCLEOSIDE ANALOGS)
PROTEASE INHIBITORS (REQUIRED FOR FINAL STAGES OF VIRUS PRODUCTION)
REVERSE TRANSCRIPTASE INHIBITORS

COMBINATION THERAPY PROLONGS LIFE AND DELAYS DISEASE PROGRESSION

PATHOGENESIS CONCEPTS

NO LATENT PHASE. CONTINUOUS VIRAL PROLIFERATION IN LYMPHOID TISSUE. LEVEL OF VIRAL RNA PARTICLES IN BLOOD CORRELATE WITH DISEASE PROGRESSION

10 BILLION VIRUS PARTICLES PRODUCED DAILY. HIGH MUTATION RATE CONTRIBUTES TO DRUG RESISTANCE

BILLIONS OF CD4 LYMPHOCYTES PRODUCED AND DESTROYED DAILY

WHEN TO TREAT

TREND IS TO EARLY TREATMENT
HIGH LEVEL VIRAL RNA IN BLOOD
FALLING CD4 COUNT. CD4 UNDER 500
SYMPTOMS OF INFECTION.

Notes

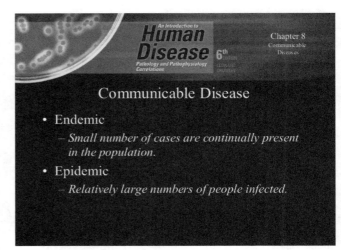

Communicable Disease

- Endemic
  - *Small number of cases are continually present in the population.*
- Epidemic
  - *Relatively large numbers of people infected.*

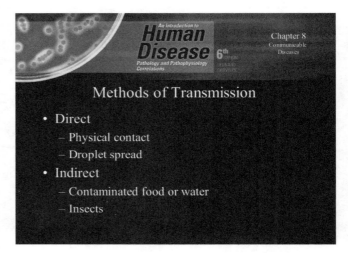

Methods of Transmission

- Direct
  - Physical contact
  - Droplet spread
- Indirect
  - Contaminated food or water
  - Insects

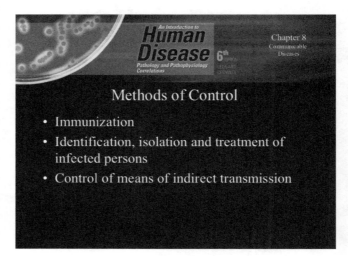

Methods of Control

- Immunization
- Identification, isolation and treatment of infected persons
- Control of means of indirect transmission

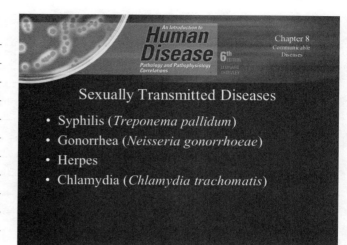

Sexually Transmitted Diseases

- Syphilis (*Treponema pallidum*)
- Gonorrhea (*Neisseria gonorrhoeae*)
- Herpes
- Chlamydia (*Chlamydia trachomatis*)

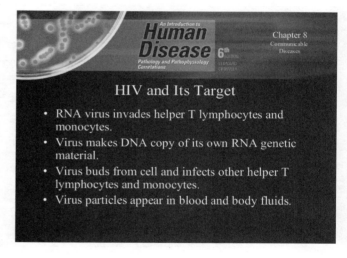

HIV and Its Target

- RNA virus invades helper T lymphocytes and monocytes.
- Virus makes DNA copy of its own RNA genetic material.
- Virus buds from cell and infects other helper T lymphocytes and monocytes.
- Virus particles appear in blood and body fluids.

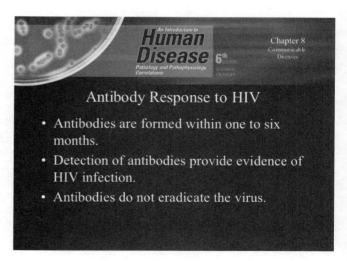

Antibody Response to HIV

- Antibodies are formed within one to six months.
- Detection of antibodies provide evidence of HIV infection.
- Antibodies do not eradicate the virus.

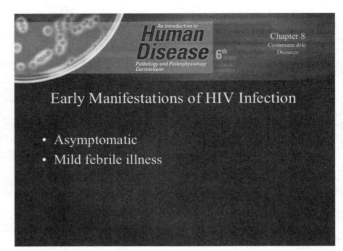

Early Manifestations of HIV Infection

- Asymptomatic
- Mild febrile illness

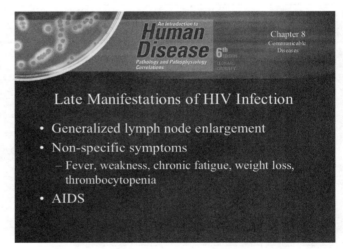

Late Manifestations of HIV Infection

- Generalized lymph node enlargement
- Non-specific symptoms
  - Fever, weakness, chronic fatigue, weight loss, thrombocytopenia
- AIDS

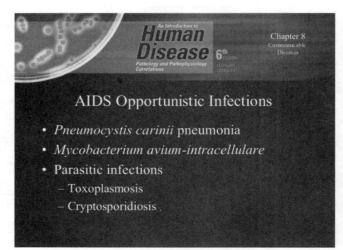

AIDS Opportunistic Infections

- *Pneumocystis carinii* pneumonia
- *Mycobacterium avium-intracellulare*
- Parasitic infections
  - Toxoplasmosis
  - Cryptosporidiosis

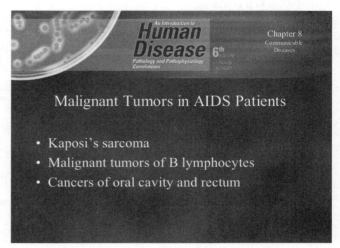

Malignant Tumors in AIDS Patients

- Kaposi's sarcoma
- Malignant tumors of B lymphocytes
- Cancers of oral cavity and rectum

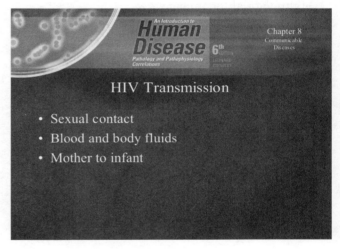

HIV Transmission

- Sexual contact
- Blood and body fluids
- Mother to infant

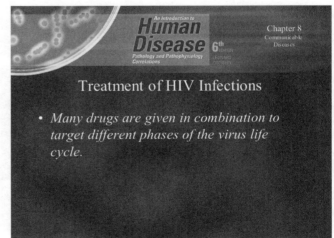

Treatment of HIV Infections

- *Many drugs are given in combination to target different phases of the virus life cycle.*

Chapter Outline

The chapter outline provides you with an organizational guide to the topics and ideas presented in this chapter of the text.

Study Questions

The following questions are provided as a test for comprehension and as a study guide for use with the text chapters. Additional study material is located at http://health.jbpub.com/humandisease/, which contains useful eLearning tools such as an A&P review, animated flashcards, interactive online glossary, crossword puzzles, and Web links.

Key Terms

Define the following terms:

1. Sex chromosome body _____

2. Chromosome nondisjunction _____

3. Chromosome translocation _____

4. Chromosome deletion _____

5. Trisomy 21 _____

Fill-in-the-Blank

1. _____ is a hereditary blood disease or condition transmitted by codominant inheritance.

2. _____ is a hereditary disease in which transmission follows an autosomal recessive inheritance pattern.

3. _____ is a hereditary disease in which transmission follows an autosomal dominant inheritance pattern.

4. _____ is a hereditary disease in which the mutant gene is transmitted on the X chromosome.

5. The incidence of congenital malformations in aborted embryos and fetuses is approximately _____.

6. Absence of chromosome 21 is called _____.

7. Most cases of Down syndrome result from _____.

True/False

Tell whether each statement is true or false. If false, explain why the statement is incorrect.

1. Some congenital abnormalities (such as congenital absence of the kidneys) may be incompatible with life after delivery. _____

    _____

2. Chromosomal abnormalities in the fetus can usually be determined by amniocentesis. _____

    _____

3. Cleft palate often results from interaction of genetic and environmental factors. _____

    _____

4. German measles acquired by the mother during pregnancy leads to *chromosomal* abnormalities in the fetus.

    _____

5. Infants born with Down syndrome usually have an extra X chromosome. _____

    _____

6. Patients born with genetically determined defects (such as phenylketonuria) have normal chromosome karyotypes.

_____

7. Fertilized ova contain 23 chromosomes. _____

_____

8. Spermatozoa usually have more chromosomes than do unfertilized ova. _____

_____

Identify

1. Identify the four main causes of congenital abnormalities.

   a. _____

   b. _____

   c. _____

   d. _____

2. Identify three maternal infections that may lead to congenital abnormalities in the fetus.

   a. _____

   b. _____

   c. _____

Matching

Match the chromosomal abnormality in the right column with the clinical condition in the left column.

1. _____ Turner syndrome   A. XXX

2. _____ Klinefelter syndrome   B. XO

3. _____ Triple X syndrome   C. Trisomy of chromosome 21

4. _____ Down syndrome   D. XXY

Discussion Questions

1. What is the difference between mitosis and meiosis? _____

   _____

   _____

   _____

2. What is the difference between a sex chromosome and an autosome? _____

   _____

   _____

   _____

3. What is a karyotype? How is it determined? _____
_____
_____

4. What is the incidence of congenital abnormalities? _____
_____
_____

5. What is the significance of a reciprocal translocation of chromosome fragments between two nonhomologous chromosomes? (*Hint:* See Case 9-1.) _____
_____
_____

6. What is Down syndrome? Under what conditions may this syndrome occur? _____
_____
_____

7. Describe the role of amniocentesis or chorionic villus sampling in the prenatal diagnosis of Down syndrome.
_____
_____
_____

8. Describe the effect of thalidomide taken by the mother on the development of the fetus. Is this drug still available?
_____
_____
_____

9. Describe how drugs are classified on the basis of possible risk to the fetus when taken by the pregnant woman.
_____
_____
_____

10. What does the term "multifactorial inheritance" mean? Give examples of diseases or conditions transmitted in this way. _____
_____
_____
_____

11. Describe the role of amniocentesis in prenatal detection of fetal abnormalities. Indicate what type of congenital abnormalities can be detected by this method, and indicate in which group of patients the method is most

widely used. _____

_____

_____

12. What methods can provide information about the number of X chromosomes possessed by an individual? _____

_____

_____

_____

13. What syndromes and conditions result from an abnormal number of sex chromosomes? _____

_____

_____

_____

14. Explain whether each of the following conditions or situations affecting the mother may lead to congenital malformations in the developing fetus.

a. Heavy cigarette smoking _____

_____

b. Heavy alcohol consumption _____

_____

c. Ingestion of a tetracycline antibiotic _____

_____

d. Penicillin tablets (Ampicillin) given to a mother to treat a urinary tract infection _____

_____

e. Dilantin taken by the mother to prevent epileptic seizures _____

_____

f. Excessive use of chewing gum _____

_____

g. Maternal infection by virus of German measles _____

_____

h. Maternal *Toxoplasma* infection _____

_____

i. Excessive consumption of egg salad sandwiches _____

_____

ABNORMALITIES IN CHROMOSOME DISTRIBUTION

SEX CHROMOSOMES
MALE XXY KLINEFELTERS
FEMALE XO TURNERS

AUTOSOMES
TRISOMY 21   DOWN'S SYNDROM
TRANSLOCATION 21

PRENATAL DIAGNOSIS
FETAL KARYOTYPE
- AMNIOCENTESIS
- CHORIONIC VILLUS SAMPLING

[BIOCHEMICAL CELL ANALYSIS]

DEVELOPMENTAL ABNORMALITIES DUE TO INTRAUTERINE INJURY

INFECTIONS	DRUGS CHEMICALS	RADIATION
GERMAN MEASLES TOXOPLASMOSIS CMV	ALCOHOL ANTICONVULSANTS MANY OTHERS—	

EFFECTS DEPEND ON STAGE OF GESTATION. MAY INVOLVE MULTIPLE ORGAN SYSTEMS.

PROTOTYPE TERATOGEN: THALIDOMIDE

CONGENITAL ABNORMALITIES

FREQUENCY: PRENATAL – SPONT. ABORTION
DETECT AT BIRTH
DETECT AFTER BIRTH

CAUSES
1. GENETIC
2. CHROMOSOMAL
   - LOSS
   - EXCESS
   - TRANSLOCATIONS – UNBALANCED
3. INTRAUTERINE INJURY
4. MULTIFACTORAL (POLYGENE)
   ENVIRONMENTAL

FDA DRUG USE IN PREGNANCY RATINGS

CATEGORY

A   NO FETAL RISK (WELL CONTROLLED STUDIES IN HUMANS)

B   NO EVIDENCE OF FETAL RISK
(ANIMAL STUDIES MAY SHOW RISK BUT HUMAN STUDIES DON'T, OR NI STUDIES IN HUMANS BUT NO RISK IN ANIMAL STUDIES)

C   CAN'T RULE OUT FETAL RISK
(NO HUMAN STUDIES AVAILABLE. ANIMAL STUDIES NOT AVAILABLE OR INDICATE POSSIBLE RISK)

D   FETAL RISK DEMONSTRATED
(DRUG NEEDED TO TREAT PATIENT. NO SAFER ALTERNATIVE. POTENTIAL BENEFIT OUTWEIGHS RISK TO FETUS

X   ABSOLUTELY CONTRAINDICATED
SEVERE RISK TO FETUS OUTWEIGHS ANY POSSIBLE BENEFIT TO PATIENT

INDICATIONS FOR AMNIOCENTESIS

MATERNAL AGE (35+)

PREVIOUS INFANT WITH
DOWN'S SYNDROME OR OTHER
CHROMOSOMAL ABNORMALITY

PARENT A TRANSLOCATION
CARRIER

OTHER CHROMOSOMAL ABNORMAL
IN EITHER PARENT

RISK OF GENETIC DISEASE IN
FETUS THAT CAN BE DETECTED
PRENATALLY

PRENATAL DIAGNOSIS

EXAMINATION OF FETAL CELLS
(AMNIOCENTESIS: EARLY 12-13 wk
LATER 14-18 wk
CHORIONIC VILLUS SAMPLING)
8-10 wk
— CHROMOSOMAL ABNORMALITIES
— BIOCHEMICAL ABNORMALITIES
— ANALYSIS OF FETAL CELL DNA

EXAMINATION OF FETAL PRODUCTS
IN AMNIONIC FLUID
⊙ ALPHA FETOPROTEIN

ULTRASOUND EXAMINATION
STRUCTURAL ABNORMALITIES
IN FETUS
○ HYDROCEPHALUS
○ ANANCEPHALY
○ URINARY TRACT ABNORMALITIES

Notes

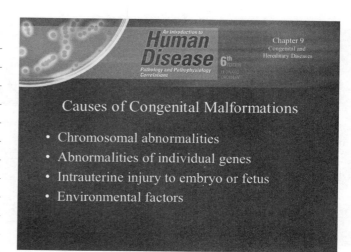

Causes of Congenital Malformations

- Chromosomal abnormalities
- Abnormalities of individual genes
- Intrauterine injury to embryo or fetus
- Environmental factors

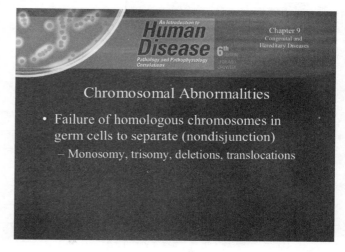

Chromosomal Abnormalities

- Failure of homologous chromosomes in germ cells to separate (nondisjunction)
  - Monosomy, trisomy, deletions, translocations

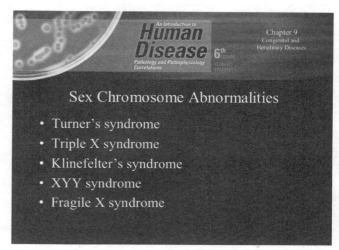

Sex Chromosome Abnormalities

- Turner's syndrome
- Triple X syndrome
- Klinefelter's syndrome
- XYY syndrome
- Fragile X syndrome

Notes

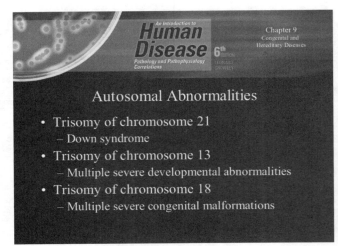

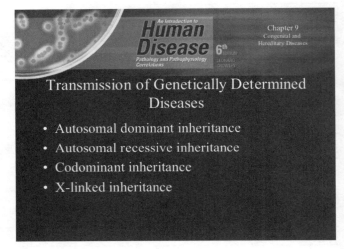

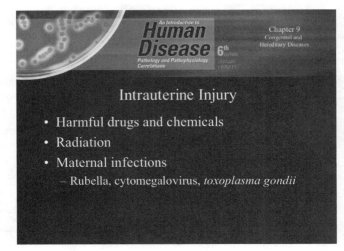

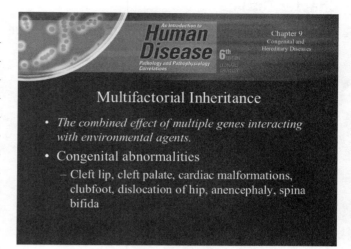

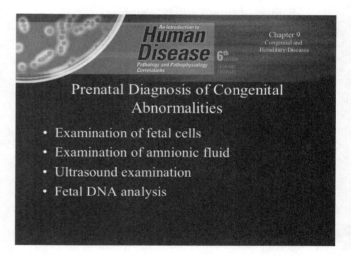

Chapter Outline

The chapter outline provides you with an organizational guide to the topics and ideas presented in this chapter of the text.

Study Questions

The following questions are provided as a test for comprehension and as a study guide for use with the text chapters. Additional study material is located at http://health.jbpub.com/humandisease/, which contains useful eLearning tools such as an A&P review, animated flashcards, interactive online glossary, crossword puzzles, and Web links.

Key Terms

Define the following terms:

1. Teratoma _____

2. Lymphoma _____

3. Precancerous condition _____

4. In situ carcinoma _____

5. Adjuvant chemotherapy _____

6. Teratoma _____

7. Nevus _____

8. Melanoma _____

9. Multiple myeloma _____

10. Leukemia _____

True/False

Tell whether each statement is true or false. If false, explain why the statement is incorrect.

1. Some neoplasms in humans may be caused by viruses. _____

   _____

2. A mutation is a cancer-causing chemical. _____

   _____

3. A Pap smear is a screening test used to detect cervical cancer. _____

   _____

4. A tumor-associated antigen is a carbohydrate protein complex secreted by tumor cells that can be used to monitor tumor growth. _____

   _____

5. A hormone-dependent tumor is one that produces sex hormones. _____

   _____

6. Anticancer drugs injure normal cells as well as cancer cells. _____

   _____

7. Adjuvant chemotherapy is used in an attempt to prevent late recurrences of cancer by destroying small foci of metastatic carcinoma before they grow to large size. _____

   _____

8. Some types of acute leukemia can be cured by chemotherapy. _____

   _____

9. Myeloma is often associated with small areas of bone destruction. _____

   _____

10. Some chemotherapy drugs impede tumor cell growth by blocking growth factor receptors on the tumor cells so that the tumor cells are unable to respond to the growth factors that stimulate cells to divide. _____

    _____

Identify

1. Give an example for each of the following:

   a. In situ carcinoma _____

   b. Teratoma _____

   c. Precancerous condition _____

2. In this list of common prefixes used to name tumors, write the meaning of the prefix after the name:

   a. Adeno _____

   b. Angio _____

   c. Chrondro _____

   d. Fibro _____

   e. Lipo _____

   f. Myo _____

   g. Neuro _____

   h. Osteo _____

   i. Lymphangio _____

   j. Hemangio _____

3. Three large groups of genes play important roles in regulating cell functions, and dysfunctions of these genes may lead to tumors. Identify these three groups of genes.

   a. _____

   b. _____

   c. _____

4. Identify four methods used to treat tumors.

   a. _____

   b. _____

   c. _____

   d. _____

5. How would you name the following neoplasms?

a. A benign tumor of fibrous connective tissue _____

b. A malignant tumor of fat cells _____

c. A benign tumor of pigment-forming cells in the skin _____

d. A neoplasm of plasma cells _____

e. A malignant tumor of mature lymphocytes _____

f. A malignant tumor of blood vessels _____

g. A malignant tumor of lymph vessels _____

h. A lymph node tumor containing many Reed-Sternberg cells _____
   _____

i. A noninfiltrating malignant tumor of cervical squamous epithelium _____
   _____

j. A malignant tumor of lymphocytes _____

k. A leukemia in which the circulating cells are immature lymphocytes _____
   _____

l. A benign tumor of the ovary composed of many different types of mature tissues _____
   _____

m. A benign tumor of cartilage _____

n. A benign pedunculated tumor arising from the epithelium of the colon _____
   _____

o. A malignant noninfiltrating tumor arising from the squamous epithelium of the cervix _____
   _____

p. A tumor of lymph nodes containing Reed-Sternberg cells intermixed with lymphocytes, plasma cells, and eosinophils _____

Discussion Questions

1. What are the major differences in growth rate, circumscription, cell differentiation, and spread between benign and malignant tumors? Give your comparison in tabular form.

	Benign Tumor	Malignant Tumor
Growth rate	_____	_____
Cell differentiation	_____	_____
Growth characteristics	_____	_____
Spread (metastasis)	_____	_____

2. Describe how tumors are named. _____

_____

_____

_____

3. What is a Pap smear? What is its application to the early diagnosis of tumors? What is the significance of a Pap smear containing atypical cells? _____

_____

_____

_____

4. What are tumor suppressor genes? What happens if one member of the pair of tumor suppressor genes fails to function normally? _____

_____

_____

_____

5. What is the Philadelphia chromosome? With what conditions is it associated? _____

_____

_____

_____

6. Describe the role of heredity in tumors. _____

_____

_____

_____

7. The eye tumor retinoblastoma is caused by mutations of both members of the paired RB genes within a single retinal cell. Explain the difference between a hereditary retinoblastoma and a sporadic retinoblastoma.

   (*Hint:* See Fig. 10-22.) _____

_____

_____

_____

8. Describe a simple classification of leukemia based on cell type and maturity of the leukemic cells. How is leukemia classified? _____

_____

_____

_____

9. How does our immune system protect us from cancer? _____

_____

_____

_____

10. What is the significance of an abnormal cervical Pap smear in a 32-year-old woman? What further diagnostic or therapeutic measures would you recommend? _____

_____

_____

_____

11. What conditions normally occur in patients with myeloma? _____

_____

_____

_____

12. A patient has a blood disease characterized by a greatly increased white blood cell count consisting of mature lymphocytes, with anemia and thrombocytopenia. What is the most likely diagnosis? _____

_____

_____

_____

TUMORS

BENIGN	MALIGNANT
MATURE CELLS	LESS DIFFERENTIATED IMMATURE
SLOW GROWTH	MORE RAPID GROWTH
EXPANSILE	INFILTRATING
LOCALIZED	METASTASES

SPREAD OF CANCER

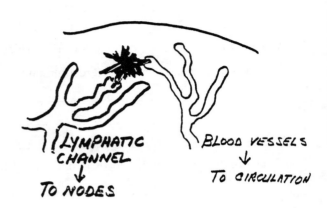

LYMPHATIC CHANNEL
↓
TO NODES

BLOOD VESSELS
↓
TO CIRCULATION

EVOLUTION OF A CANCER

NORMAL EPITHELIUM

ALTERED EPITHELIUM MILD MODERATE MARKED

IN SITU CARCINOMA

INFILTRATING CARCINOMA

PRECANCEROUS CONDITION - SOME CASES WILL EVOLVE INTO CANCER

TERMINOLOGY

BENIGN
1. DESCRIPTIVE — POLYP. PAPILLOMA
2. TISSUE OF ORIGIN + OMA
   FIBROMA   CHONDROMA
   OSTEOMA   ANGIOMA
   MYOMA
   ADENOMA

MALIGNANT

EPITHELIUM (SURFACE-GLANDS-ORGANS) CARCINOMA

CONNECTIVE AND SUPPORTING SARCOMA

BLOOD CELLS LEUKEMIA

TERMINOLOGY EXCEPTIONS

LYMPHOMA

TERATOMA

TUMORS OF MELANIN PIGMENT
    PRODUCING CELLS
        BENIGN: NEVUS ("MOLE")
        MALIGNANT: MELANOMA
                ("BLACK CANCER")

PRIMITIVE CELL TUMORS

DIAGNOSIS-MANAGEMENT

1. AN ABNORMALITY OF FORM
   OR FUNCTION
   (BUT DON'T WAIT FOR THIS)*

2. EXAMINATION

3. BIOPSY OR EXCISION

4. CONSIDER OPTIONS AND
   CHOOSE TREATMENT

   *SCREENING
    PAP. SMEAR
    MAMMOGRAMS
    PROSTATIC ANTIGEN IN BLOOD
    STOOL EXAM FOR BLOOD

RECOGNITION OF TUMORS

GROSS APPEARANCE
MICROSCOPIC APPEARANCE

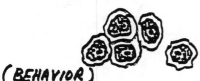

(BEHAVIOR)

CLASSIFICATION OF TUMORS

PROGNOSIS - MANAGEMENT
IMPLICATIONS

HEREDITY AND TUMORS

MULTIFACTORIAL
    SETS OF GENES INHERITED THAT
    AFFECT CELL FUNCTION AND SLIGHTLY
    INCREASE SUSCEPTIBILITY TO SOME
    TUMORS

INDIVIDUAL GENE MUTATIONS
• INHERITED NON FUNCTIONAL TUMOR
  SUPPRESSOR GENE (GERMLINE
  MUTATION) IN ALL CELLS
• RANDOM MUTATION OF SECOND TUMOR
  SUPPRESSOR GENE IN A SINGLE
  CELL DEREGULATES CELL

OTHER FACTORS LEADING TO TUMORS

VIRUSES: LYMPHOMA-LEUKEMIA VIRUS
         PAPILLOMA VIRUS, EB VIRUS,
         HBV, HCV,
CHROMOSOME ABNORMALITIES: S.G.
                PHILADELPHIA CHROMOSOME

FAILURE OF IMMUNOLOGIC DEFENSES:
         AIDS
         IMMUNOSUPPRESSION

TREATMENT

BENIGN
EXCISE (OR DO NOTHING)
PRECANCEROUS EXCISE

MALIGNANT
SURGERY
RADIOTHERAPY
HORMONES
    SEX HORMONES
    CORTICOSTEROIDS
ANTICANCER DRUGS
    BLOCK: DNA → RNA → PROTEIN → CELL
                       SYNTHESIS DIVISION

ADJUVANT CHEMOTHERAPY
IMMUNOTHERAPY
ROLE OF TUMOR MARKERS

PATHOGENESIS OF TUMORS

GENE MUTATIONS DISRUPT NORMAL CELL FUNCTIONS

TARGET GENES	MALFUNCTION
PROTO-ONCOGENES PROMOTE CELL GROWTH	POINT MUTATION AMPLIFICATION TRANSLOCATION
PAIRED TUMOR SUPPRESSOR GENES (ON HOMOLOGOUS CHROMOSOMES) INHIBIT CELL PROLIFERATION	BOTH GENES INACTIVATED BY MUTATIONS IN THE SAME CELL
MUTATOR GENES CORRECT ERRORS IN DNA DUPLICATION	MUTATION RATE INCREASED

"GERMLINE" MUTATION OF SUPPRESSOR GENES AND SUSCEPTIBILITY TO TUMORS

GERMLINE MUTATION

INHERITED NON FUNCTIONAL TS GENE IN ALL CELLS

ACQUIRED MUTATION OF REMAINING FUNCTIONAL TS GENE IN SINGLE CELL

NO FUNCTIONING TS GENES IN AFFECTED CELL

SPORADIC MUTATION

TWO NORMAL TS GENES IN ALL CELLS

SPONTANEOUS MUTATION OF ONE TS GENE IN SINGLE CELL

SECOND SPONTANEOUS MUTATION OF TS GENE IN SAME CELL

LOSS OF TS CONTROL FUNCTION IN AFFECTED CELL

CLONE OF IDENTICAL DEREGULATED CELLS

TUMOR

THE PHILADELPHIA CHROMOSOME
CHROMOSOMES 9-22 RECIPROCAL TRANSLOCATIONS

CHROMOSOME 9

CHROMOSOME 22

BCR GENE
SITE OF BREAK

PROTOONCOGENE ABL

SITE OF BREAK

PHILADELPHIA CHROMOSOME

COMPOSITE GENE (ABL/BCR) CODES FOR PROTEIN THAT STIMULATES EXCESS WHITE BLOOD CELL PROLIFERATION

IMMUNOTHERAPY CONCEPTS

CYTOTOXIC T CELLS (T8) RECOGNIZE TUMOR ANTIGENS PRESENTED WITH MHC CLASS I ANTIGENS AND ATTACK TUMOR CELLS

NK CELLS ATTACK TUMOR CELLS

ACTIVATED MACROPHAGES ATTACK AND DESTROY TUMOR CELLS BY PHAGOCYTOSIS AND CYTOKINES, AND ATTRACT OTHER DESTRUCTIVE CELLS

ANTIBODIES AGAINST TUMOR CELLS DESTROY TUMOR CELLS VIA COMPLEMENT ACTIVATION

IMMUNOTHERAPY TREATMENT

NONSPECIFIC
- CYTOKINES, INTERFERONS, INTERLEUKIN-2 AND OTHERS

SPECIFIC
- TUMOR INFILTRATING LYMPHOCYTES
- TUMOR VACCINES
- TUMOR ANTIBODIES

CONCEPT OF MULTISTEP PROGRESSION OF GENETIC CHANGES LEADING TO TUMORS

GENETIC CHANGE GIVES CELL A GROWTH ADVANTAGE

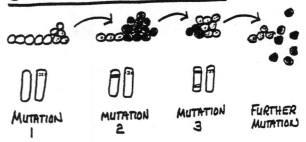

MUTATION 1   MUTATION 2   MUTATION 3   FURTHER MUTATION

CONCEPT OF UNSTABLE TUMOR GENOME
AMPLIFICATIONS
DELETIONS
TRANSLOCATIONS

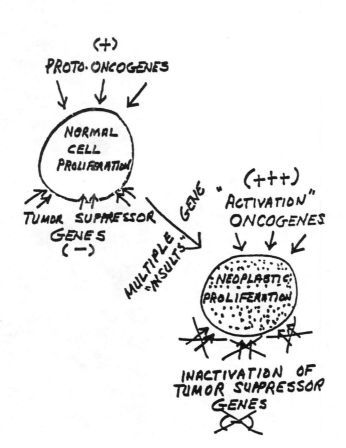

(+)
PROTO-ONCOGENES

NORMAL CELL PROLIFERATION

TUMOR SUPPRESSOR GENES (−)

MULTIPLE "INSULTS" GENE

(+++) "ACTIVATION" ONCOGENES

NEOPLASTIC PROLIFERATION

INACTIVATION OF TUMOR SUPPRESSOR GENES

Notes

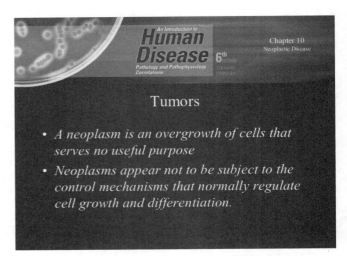

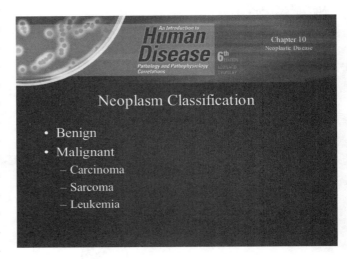

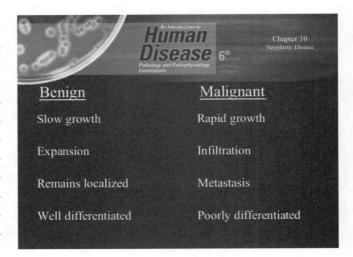

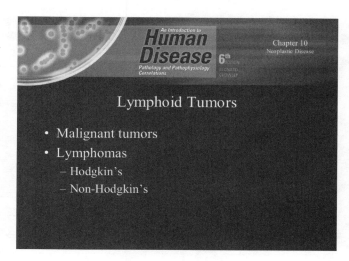

Chapter 10
Neoplastic Disease

Lymphoid Tumors

- Malignant tumors
- Lymphomas
  - Hodgkin's
  - Non-Hodgkin's

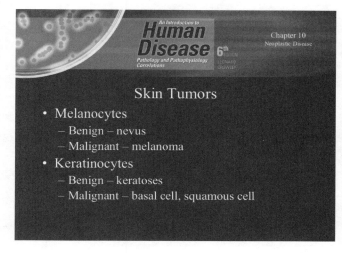

Chapter 10
Neoplastic Disease

Skin Tumors

- Melanocytes
  - Benign – nevus
  - Malignant – melanoma
- Keratinocytes
  - Benign – keratoses
  - Malignant – basal cell, squamous cell

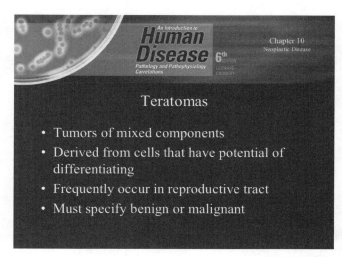

Chapter 10
Neoplastic Disease

Teratomas

- Tumors of mixed components
- Derived from cells that have potential of differentiating
- Frequently occur in reproductive tract
- Must specify benign or malignant

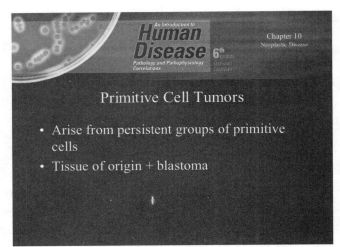

Primitive Cell Tumors

- Arise from persistent groups of primitive cells
- Tissue of origin + blastoma

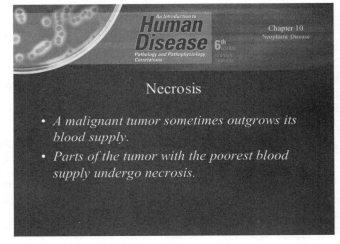

Necrosis

- *A malignant tumor sometimes outgrows its blood supply.*
- *Parts of the tumor with the poorest blood supply undergo necrosis.*

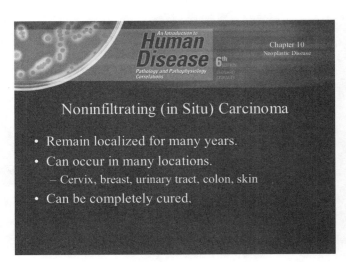

Noninfiltrating (in Situ) Carcinoma

- Remain localized for many years.
- Can occur in many locations.
  - Cervix, breast, urinary tract, colon, skin
- Can be completely cured.

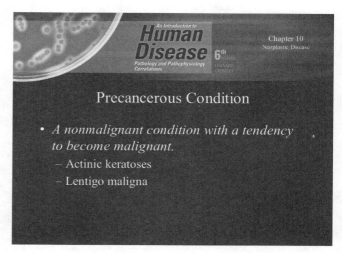

Precancerous Condition

- *A nonmalignant condition with a tendency to become malignant.*
  - Actinic keratoses
  - Lentigo maligna

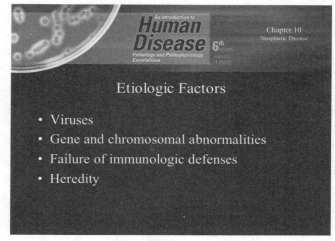

Etiologic Factors

- Viruses
- Gene and chromosomal abnormalities
- Failure of immunologic defenses
- Heredity

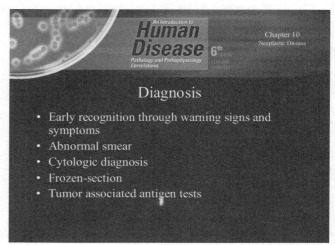

Diagnosis

- Early recognition through warning signs and symptoms
- Abnormal smear
- Cytologic diagnosis
- Frozen-section
- Tumor associated antigen tests

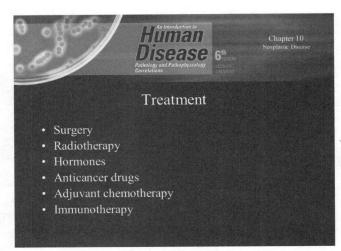

Treatment

- Surgery
- Radiotherapy
- Hormones
- Anticancer drugs
- Adjuvant chemotherapy
- Immunotherapy

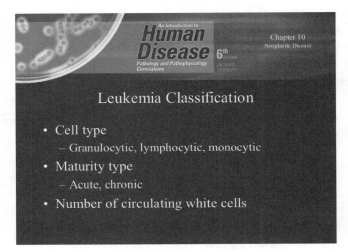

Leukemia Classification

- Cell type
  - Granulocytic, lymphocytic, monocytic
- Maturity type
  - Acute, chronic
- Number of circulating white cells

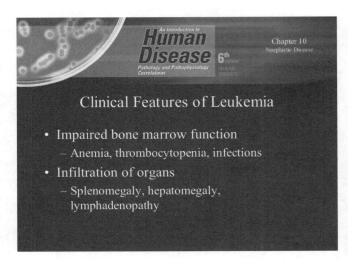

Clinical Features of Leukemia

- Impaired bone marrow function
  - Anemia, thrombocytopenia, infections
- Infiltration of organs
  - Splenomegaly, hepatomegaly, lymphadenopathy

Notes

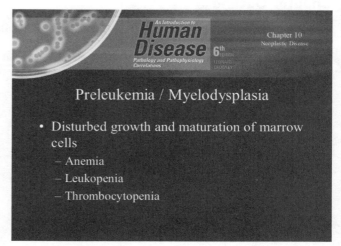

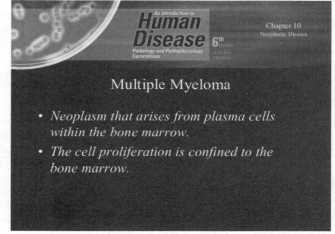

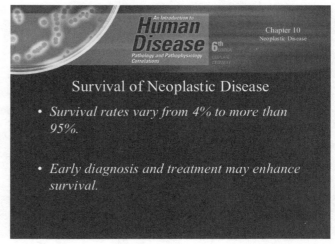

Chapter Outline

The chapter outline provides you with an organizational guide to the topics and ideas presented in this chapter of the text.

Hemostasis
Factors Concerned with Hemostasis
    Blood Vessels and Platelets
    Plasma Coagulation Factors
    Coagulation Inhibitors and Fibrinolysins
    Calcium and Blood Coagulation
Clinical Disturbances of Blood Coagulation
    Abnormalities of Small Blood Vessels
    Abnormalities of Platelet Numbers or Function
    Deficiency of Plasma Coagulation Factors
    Liberation of Thromboplastic Material into the Circulation
    Relative Frequency of Various Coagulation Disturbances
Laboratory Tests to Evaluate Hemostasis
Case Studies

Study Questions

The following questions are provided as a test for comprehension and as a study guide for use with the text chapters. Additional study material is located at http://health.jbpub.com/humandisease/, which contains useful eLearning tools such as an A&P review, animated flashcards, interactive online glossary, crossword puzzles, and Web links.

Key Terms

Define the following terms:

1. Hemostasis _____

2. Platelets _____

3. Blood coagulation _____

4. Hemophilia A _____

5. Von Willebrand's disease _____

6. Thrombocytopenia _____

7. Hemorrhage _____

8. Coagulation factors _____

9. Thromboplastin _____

Identify

1. Identify the four factors required for normal hemostasis.

a. _____

b. _____

c. _____

d. _____

Discussion Questions

1. Construct a simple system to describe the sequence of events involved in normal blood coagulation. (*Hint:* See Fig. 11-1.)

2. Describe the role of platelets in blood coagulation. _____

_____

_____

_____

3. Describe the characteristic appearance of the bleeding associated with platelet deficiency. _____

_____

_____

_____

4. Describe the differences between hemophilia A and von Willebrand's disease. _____

_____

_____

_____

5. What is the disseminated intravascular coagulation syndrome? _____

_____

_____

_____

6. What factors initiate the disseminated intravascular coagulation syndrome? _____

_____

_____

_____

7. List some of the readily available laboratory tests commonly used to evaluate the functions of the various factors involved in blood coagulation. Indicate what each test measures. _____

_____

_____

_____

_____

8. What is the consequence of liberation of thromboplastic material into the circulation? _____

_____

_____

_____

9. What types of diseases produce abnormalities in the first phase of blood coagulation? _____

_____

_____

_____

10. What conditions lead to disturbances in the second phase of blood coagulation? _____

_____

_____

_____

11. What types of diseases are associated with thrombocytopenia? _____

_____

_____

_____

12. What are the major types of blood coagulations? _____

_____

_____

_____

13. A five-year-old male child experiences frequent areas of hemorrhage into joints and muscles following minor trauma. Laboratory tests reveal a reduced concentration of a plasma coagulation factor that is concerned with the early stage of the coagulation mechanism (formation of thromboplastin). What is the most likely diagnosis?

_____

_____

_____

HEMOSTATIC MECHANISMS

BLOOD VESSELS
PLATELETS
PLASMA COAGULATION FACTORS
FIBRINOLYSINS AND INHIBITORS
CALCIUM IONS (CA^{2+})

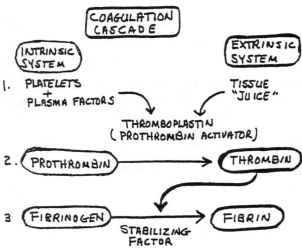

COAGULATION CASCADE

INTRINSIC SYSTEM   EXTRINSIC SYSTEM

1. PLATELETS
   +
   PLASMA FACTORS   TISSUE "JUICE"

   THROMBOPLASTIN
   (PROTHROMBIN ACTIVATOR)

2. PROTHROMBIN ──→ THROMBIN

3. FIBRINOGEN ──→ FIBRIN
   STABILIZING FACTOR

FIBRINOLYSIS

THE CLOTTING PROCESS SIMULTANEOUSLY GENERATES MECHANISMS TO CONTROL CLOTTING

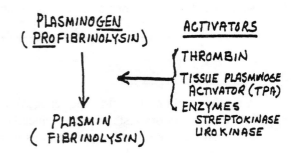

PLASMINOGEN (PROFIBRINOLYSIN)

ACTIVATORS
  THROMBIN
  TISSUE PLASMINOGE ACTIVATOR (TPA)
  ENZYMES
    STREPTOKINASE
    UROKINASE

PLASMIN (FIBRINOLYSIN)

CLINICAL APPLICATIONS: "CLOTBUSTERS"
          STROKES
          HEART ATTACKS

COAGULATION PROBLEMS

FIRST PHASE

   INADEQUATE PLATELETS

      INADEQUATE PRODUCTION: BONE MARROW DISEASE
      EXCESSIVE DESTRUCTION: AUTOIMMUNE DISEASE

   COAGULATION FACTOR DEFICIENCY: HEREDITARY

      CLASSIC HEMOPHILIA (HEMOPHILIA A) FACTOR VIII
      CHRISTMAS DISEASE (HEMOPHILIA B) FACTOR IX
      VON WILLEBRAND'S DISEASE (VON W. FACTOR)

SECOND PHASE: MOST ARE ACQUIRED
   FACTORS MADE IN LIVER AND REQUIRE
   VITAMIN K FOR SYNTHESIS [FAT SOL.
   VITAMIN. COUMADIN ANTICOAGULANTS
   BLOCK FUNCTION OF VITAMIN

   PROBLEMS

NO INTESTINAL BACTERIA	ANTIBIOTICS
NO BILE IN INTESTINE	BLOCKED BILE DUCT
DRUGS BLOCK ACTION	COUMADIN
DAMAGED LIVER CAN'T MAKE FACTORS	LIVER DISEASE

COMMON PROBLEM: DISSEMINATED INTRAVASCULAR COAGULATION

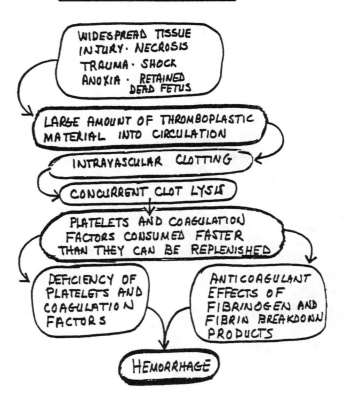

WIDESPREAD TISSUE INJURY· NECROSIS TRAUMA· SHOCK ANOXIA · RETAINED DEAD FETUS

LARGE AMOUNT OF THROMBOPLASTIC MATERIAL INTO CIRCULATION

INTRAVASCULAR CLOTTING

CONCURRENT CLOT LYSIS

PLATELETS AND COAGULATION FACTORS CONSUMED FASTER THAN THEY CAN BE REPLENISHED

DEFICIENCY OF PLATELETS AND COAGULATION FACTORS

ANTICOAGULANT EFFECTS OF FIBRINOGEN AND FIBRIN BREAKDOWN PRODUCTS

HEMORRHAGE

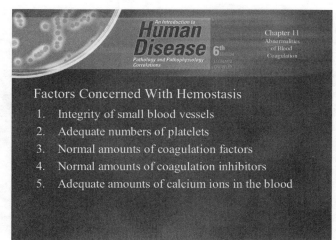

Factors Concerned With Hemostasis

1. Integrity of small blood vessels
2. Adequate numbers of platelets
3. Normal amounts of coagulation factors
4. Normal amounts of coagulation inhibitors
5. Adequate amounts of calcium ions in the blood

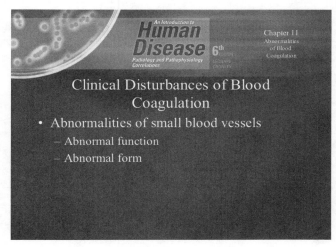

Clinical Disturbances of Blood Coagulation

- Abnormalities of small blood vessels
  - Abnormal function
  - Abnormal form

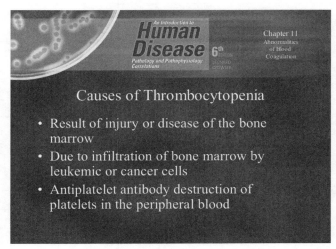

Causes of Thrombocytopenia

- Result of injury or disease of the bone marrow
- Due to infiltration of bone marrow by leukemic or cancer cells
- Antiplatelet antibody destruction of platelets in the peripheral blood

Notes

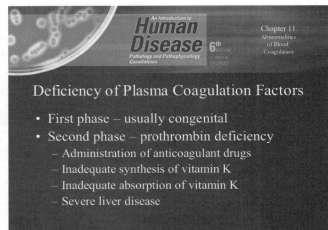

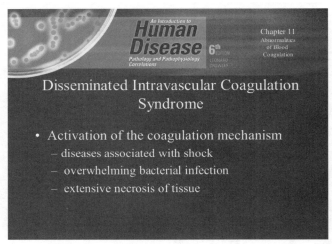

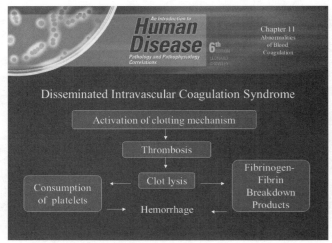

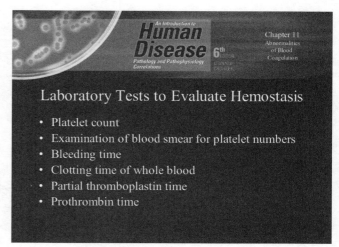

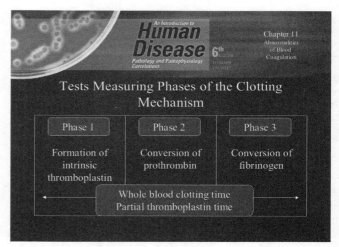

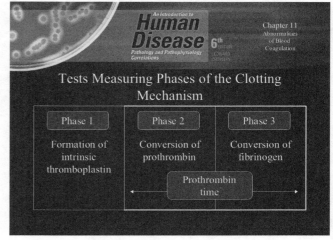

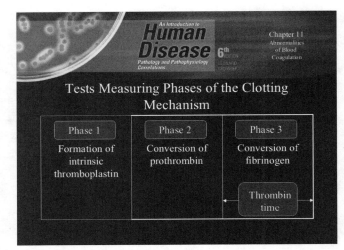

Chapter 12   Circulatory Disturbances

Chapter Outline

The chapter outline provides you with an organizational guide to the topics and ideas presented in this chapter of the text.

Study Questions

The following questions are provided as a test for comprehension and as a study guide for use with the text chapters. Additional study material is located at http://health.jbpub.com/humandisease/, which contains useful eLearning tools such as an A&P review, animated flashcards, interactive online glossary, crossword puzzles, and Web links.

Key Terms

Define the following terms:

1. Edema _____

2. Thrombus _____

3. Embolus _____

4. Infarct _____

Fill-in-the-Blank

1. Reduced capillary osmotic pressure can be caused by _____.

2. Increased capillary permeability can be caused by _____.

3. _____ results in increased capillary hydrostatic pressure.

4. _____ results in obstruction of lymphatic channels.

5. If the capillary hydrostatic pressure exceeds the osmotic pressure, _____ will result.

True/False

Tell whether each of the following statements is true or false. If false, explain why the statement is incorrect.

1. Rapid release of thromboplastic material into the circulation activates the blood coagulation and fibrinolytic systems, and leads to a disseminated intravascular coagulation syndrome. _____

   _____

2. Slow release of thromboplastic material into the circulation activates the blood coagulation and fibrinolytic systems, and leads to a disseminated intravascular coagulation syndrome. _____

   _____

3. Slow release of thromboplastic material into the circulation activates the blood coagulation and fibrinolytic systems but also causes a compensatory increase in platelets and blood proteins concerned with blood coagulation (coagulation factors), which predisposes the person to intravascular thromboses. _____

   _____

4. Formation of blood clots within leg veins results primarily from slowing or stasis of blood in leg veins. _____

   _____

5. A large pulmonary embolus that completely blocks both pulmonary arteries causes infarction of both lungs.

   _____

Identify

1. Identify the four main causes of edema.

   a. _____

   b. _____

   c. _____

   d. _____

2. Identify the three conditions that may lead to the formation of blood clots within the heart.

   a. _____

   b. _____

   c. _____

3. Identify three diagnostic measures that may assist the clinician in making the diagnosis of a pulmonary infarct.

   a. _____

   b. _____

   c. _____

Matching

Several factors predispose to the formation of blood clots within blood vessels:

A. Sluggish blood flow within a blood vessel
B. Damage to the wall of a blood vessel
C. Increased coagulability of the blood

Write the letter of the factor that is of greatest importance in the following situations next to each statement.

1. _____ A thrombus formed in a coronary artery in which the lining (intima) is roughened by accumulation of cholesterol and other lipids in the arterial wall

2. _____ A thrombus formed in an artery of a healthy young woman taking birth control pills

3. _____ A thrombus in a leg vein of a healthy middle-aged man who had recently completed a 10-hour nonstop airplane flight

Discussion Questions

1. What factors regulate the flow of fluid into and out of the capillaries? (*Hint:* See Fig. 12-9.) _____

   _____

   _____

   _____

2. Why do some patients with cancer develop blood clots within their circulation because they have a higher-than-normal level of platelets and blood coagulation factors? _____

   _____

   _____

   _____

3. What is the difference between a thrombus and an embolus? _____

   _____

   _____

   _____

4. What factors predispose a person to venous thrombosis? What are the major complications of a thrombus in a

   leg vein? _____

   _____

   _____

   _____

5. What factors predispose a person to arterial thrombosis? _____

   _____

   _____

   _____

6. What conditions predispose a person to thrombosis by increasing the coagulability of the blood? _____

   _____

   _____

   _____

7. What is the usual source of pulmonary emboli? _____

   _____

   _____

   _____

8. A six-year-old child has marked edema of the legs and edema fluid within the abdominal cavity (ascites). The
   child's blood protein and albumin levels are much lower than normal. The urine contains large amounts of protein.

   What is the most likely cause of the edema? _____

   _____

   _____

   _____

9. A 58-year-old woman sustains a large pulmonary embolus that completely blocks the main pulmonary artery.
   Explain whether each of the following descriptors applies to the condition. Why or why not?

   a. Patient experiences severe pleuritic chest pain _____

   _____

   b. Patient becomes short of breath _____

   _____

c. Lung scan is abnormal _____

_____

d. Chest X-ray is abnormal _____

_____

e. Patient had pulmonary infarct _____

_____

f. Patient coughs up blood _____

_____

10. What populations have a greater-than-normal risk of developing thromboembolic disease? _____

_____

_____

_____

11. What factors predispose a person to postoperative venous thromboses? _____

_____

_____

_____

12. What conditions may result from a blood clot that forms in the left ventricle after a myocardial infarction? _____

_____

_____

_____

THROMBOSIS

CAUSES
LOCAL—
   STASIS
   INJURY TO VESSEL WALL
   (SMOOTH ENDOTHELIUM DISRUPTED)
SYSTEMIC—
   INCREASED COAGULABILITY OF BLOOD
   — POSTOPERATIVE
   — THE "PILL"

LOCATION

ARTERIAL
   BRAIN
   HEART
   EXTREMETIES

VENOUS

COMPLICATION

INFARCTION

PULMONARY EMBOLISM
   LARGE- OBSTRUCT
       PULMONARY
       BLOOD FLOW
   SMALL- INFARCT
       OF LUNG

PULMONARY ARTERY

ALVEOLAR   PULM.
CAPILLARIES   VEINS

BRONCHIAL ARTERY

EMBOLISM: COLLATERAL FLOW FROM BRONCHIAL ARTERIES

EMBOLISM: INSUFFICIENT COLLATERAL FLOW = INFARCT

INTRACARDIAC THROMBI

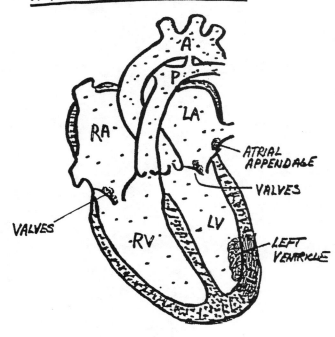

A
P
RA
LA
ATRIAL APPENDAGE
VALVES
VALVES
RV
LV
LEFT VENTRICLE

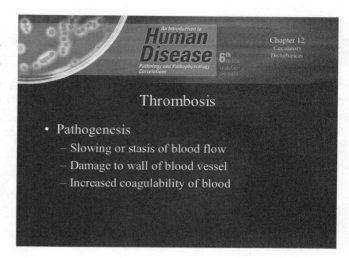

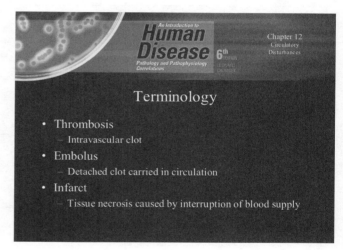

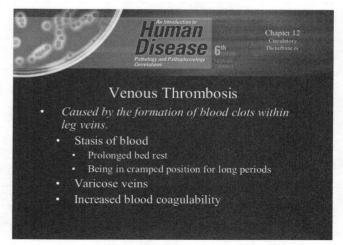

Notes

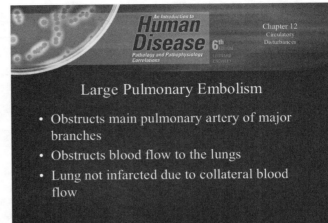

Large Pulmonary Embolism

- Obstructs main pulmonary artery of major branches
- Obstructs blood flow to the lungs
- Lung not infarcted due to collateral blood flow

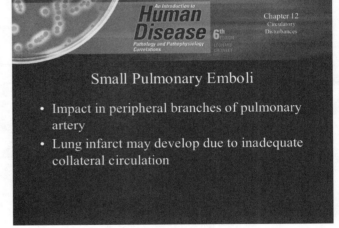

Small Pulmonary Emboli

- Impact in peripheral branches of pulmonary artery
- Lung infarct may develop due to inadequate collateral circulation

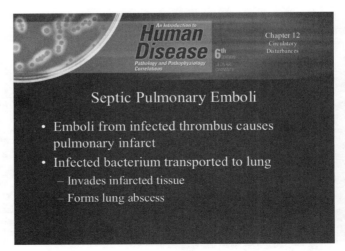

Septic Pulmonary Emboli

- Emboli from infected thrombus causes pulmonary infarct
- Infected bacterium transported to lung
  - Invades infarcted tissue
  - Forms lung abscess

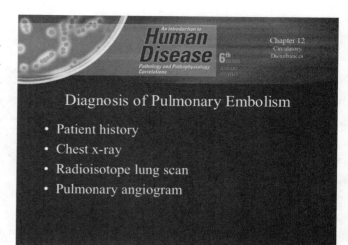

Diagnosis of Pulmonary Embolism

- Patient history
- Chest x-ray
- Radioisotope lung scan
- Pulmonary angiogram

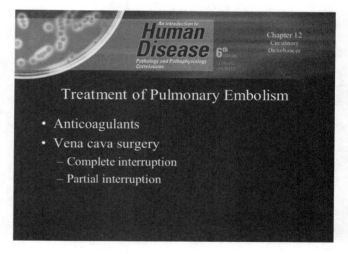

Treatment of Pulmonary Embolism

- Anticoagulants
- Vena cava surgery
  - Complete interruption
  - Partial interruption

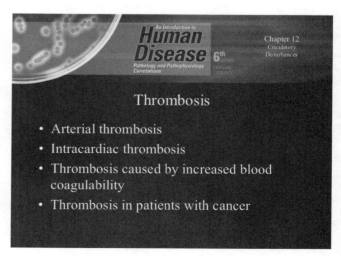

Thrombosis

- Arterial thrombosis
- Intracardiac thrombosis
- Thrombosis caused by increased blood coagulability
- Thrombosis in patients with cancer

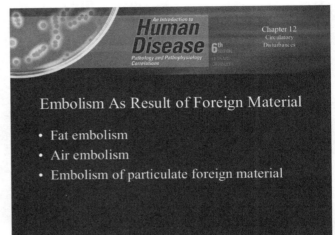

Embolism As Result of Foreign Material

- Fat embolism
- Air embolism
- Embolism of particulate foreign material

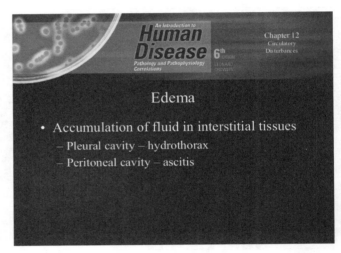

Edema

- Accumulation of fluid in interstitial tissues
  - Pleural cavity – hydrothorax
  - Peritoneal cavity – ascitis

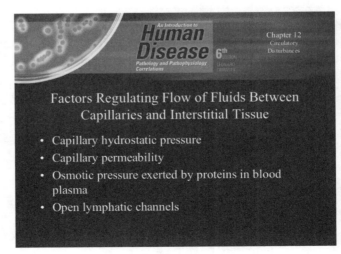

Factors Regulating Flow of Fluids Between Capillaries and Interstitial Tissue

- Capillary hydrostatic pressure
- Capillary permeability
- Osmotic pressure exerted by proteins in blood plasma
- Open lymphatic channels

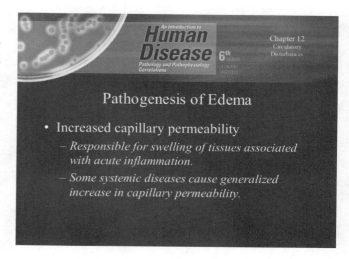

Pathogenesis of Edema

- Increased capillary permeability
  - *Responsible for swelling of tissues associated with acute inflammation.*
  - *Some systemic diseases cause generalized increase in capillary permeability.*

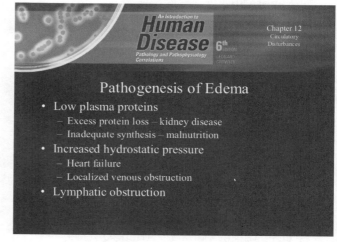

Pathogenesis of Edema

- Low plasma proteins
  - Excess protein loss – kidney disease
  - Inadequate synthesis – malnutrition
- Increased hydrostatic pressure
  - Heart failure
  - Localized venous obstruction
- Lymphatic obstruction

Chapter Outline

The chapter outline provides you with an organizational guide to the topics and ideas presented in this chapter of the text.

Cardiac Structure and Function
Normal Cardiac Function
    Cardiac Chambers
    Cardiac Valves
    Blood Supply to the Heart
    Conduction System of the Heart
    Blood Pressure
Heart Disease as a Disturbance of Pump Function
Congenital Heart Disease
    Prevention of Congenital Heart Disease
Valvular Heart Disease
    Rheumatic Fever and Rheumatic Heart Disease
    Nonrheumatic Aortic Stenosis
    Mitral Valve Prolapse
    Serotonin-Related Heart Valve Damage
    Infective Endocarditis
Coronary Heart Disease
    Risk Factors
    Manifestations and Complications
Myocardial Infarction
    Location of Myocardial Infarcts
    Complications of Myocardial Infarcts
    Survival After Myocardial Infarction
    Diagnosis of Myocardial Infarction
    Treatment of Myocardial Infarction
Case Studies
Coronary Artery Disease
    Diagnosis of Coronary Artery Disease
    Treatment of Coronary Artery Disease
    Taking Aspirin to Reduce Risk of Cardiovascular Disease
    Cocaine-Induced Arrhythmias and Myocardial Infarcts
    Blood Lipids and Coronary Artery Disease
    Homocysteine and Cardiovascular Disease
    Chlamydia pneumoniae and Cardiovascular Disease
Hypertension and Hypertensive Cardiovascular Disease
    Cardiac Effects
    Vascular Effects
    Renal Effects
    Cause and Treatment of Hypertension

Primary Myocardial Disease
   Myocarditis
   Cardiomyopathy
Heart Failure
Acute Pulmonary Edema
Aneurysms
   Arteriosclerotic Aneurysm
   Dissecting Aneurysm of the Aorta
Diseases of the Veins
   Venous Thrombosis and Thrombophlebitis
   Varicose Veins of the Lower Extremities
   Varicose Veins in Other Locations

Study Questions

The following questions are provided as a test for comprehension and as a study guide for use with the text chapters. Additional study material is located at http://health.jbpub.com/humandisease/, which contains useful eLearning tools such as an A&P review, animated flashcards, interactive online glossary, crossword puzzles, and Web links.

Key Terms

Define the following terms:

1. Bacterial endocarditis _____

2. Disecting aneurysm _____

3. Stent _____

4. Atherosclerosis _____

5. Rheumatic fever _____

6. Arteriosclerotic aneurysm _____

7. Angina pectoris _____

8. Myocardial infarction _____

9. Lipoprotein _____

Fill-in-the-Blank

1. The _____ valves are open in systole.

2. The _____ valves are open in diastole.

3. A dissecting aneurysm of the aorta is due to _____.

4. One of the important complications of mitral valve scarring due to rheumatic fever is _____.

5. The _____ stage in the formation of an atheromatous plaque is reversible.

True/False

Tell whether each statement is true or false. If false, explain why the statement is incorrect.

1. A coronary artery narrowed by an atheromatous plaque often can be dilated successfully by coronary angioplasty.

   _____

2. A successfully dilated coronary artery may undergo restenosis, but using a stent to keep the vessel open reduces the incidence of restenosis. _____

   _____

3. Stents coated with drugs that suppress the cell proliferation responsible for the restenosis have not been effective and are not recommended to prevent restenosis. _____

   _____

4. The left anterior descending coronary artery supplies the back wall of the heart. _____

   _____

5. Impulses that cause the heart to beat are initiated in the sinoatrial (SA) node. _____

_____

6. The systolic pressure is a measure of the resistance to blood flow due to constriction of the peripheral arterioles.

_____

7. The rate of flow through arteries varies directly with the radius of the artery. _____

_____

Identify

1. Identify the four major factors that are known to increase the risk of coronary heart disease.

   a. _____

   b. _____

   c. _____

   d. _____

2. Identify five complications of an acute myocardial infarction.

   a. _____

   b. _____

   c. _____

   d. _____

   e. _____

3. The term "acute coronary syndrome" includes three different conditions. What are they?

   a. _____

   b. _____

   c. _____

Discussion Questions

1. Describe how heart valves function to provide unidirectional flow of blood through the heart. _____

_____

_____

_____

2. Describe what happens if the mitral valve doesn't open properly, and what happens if it doesn't close properly.

_____

_____

_____

3. What are the structural changes in the mitral valve that lead to mitral valve prolapse? _____

_____

_____

_____

4. What factors predispose a person to calcific aortic stenosis? _____

_____

_____

_____

5. Describe the conditions that predispose a person to infective endocarditis. _____

_____

_____

_____

6. Which patients should have antibiotic prophylaxis prior to dental procedures or surgical procedures? _____

_____

_____

_____

7. What types of diets lower blood lipids? _____

_____

_____

_____

8. Describe the effect on cardiovascular function resulting from damage to a mitral valve papillary muscle as a result of a myocardial infarction. _____

_____

_____

_____

9. Why are cardiac enzyme tests performed on the blood of patients suspected of having a myocardial infarction?

_____

_____

_____

10. A patient complains of chest pain. Clinical examination, enzyme tests, and electrocardiogram reveal a thrombosis of the left anterior descending coronary artery. How should the patient be treated? _____

_____

_____

_____

11. What methods can be used to reestablish blood flow through a blocked coronary artery? _____

_____

_____

_____

12. Describe the effect of high blood pressure on the heart and vascular system. _____

_____

_____

_____

13. Patients at risk for coronary heart disease frequently take low-dose aspirin tablets daily to reduce the risk of heart attacks. What effect does aspirin have? Why is it used? _____

_____

_____

_____

14. What conditions may lead to cardiac valve scarring? _____

_____

_____

_____

15. What conditions may follow a myocardial infarction? _____

_____

_____

_____

16. What diagnostic measures may assist the clinician in making a diagnosis of acute myocardial infarction? _____

_____

_____

_____

17. What is the cause of an aneurysm of the abdominal aorta that occurs in an elderly individual? How is it treated?

_____

_____

_____

18. What happens during congestive cardiac failure? _____

_____

_____

_____

19. What conditions may cause mitral insufficiency? _____

_____

_____

_____

20. What is C-reactive protein (CRP)? What does an elevated CRP test indicate? _____

_____

_____

_____

HEART DISEASE

FAULTY CONSTRUCTION	CONGENITAL
MALFUNCTIONING VALVES	VALVULAR
FUEL LINE PROBLEMS	CORONARY
OVERLOADED PUMP	HYPERTENSIVE
MALFUNCTIONING PUMP	PRIMARY MYOCARDIAL DISEASE

VALVE INFECTIONS
(INFECTIVE ENDOCARDITIS)

MICRO-ORGANISMS IMPLANT ON VALVE → VALVE DESTRUCTION

↓

INFECTED EMBOLI

PERSONS AT RISK
ABNORMAL VALVES
INTRAVENOUS DRUG ABUSERS

TREATMENT
ANTIBIOTICS
VALVE REPLACEMENT

VALVULAR HEART DISEASE

AORTIC STENOSIS CAUSED BY VALVE CALCIFICATION
OF NORMAL VALVE LEAFLETS
OF BICUSPID AORTIC VALVE

MITRAL VALVE PROLAPSE
ISOLATED PROLAPSE WITHOUT REGURGITATION
PROLAPSE WITH REGURGITATION

VALVE DAMAGED CAUSED BY RHEUMATIC FEVER

VALVE DAMAGE CAUSED BY SEROTONIN OR
SIMILAR SUBSTANCES

MITRAL VALVE PROLAPSE

RHEUMATIC VALVE DISEASE
BICUSPID AORTIC VALVE

CALCIFIC AORTIC VALVE

FUEL LINE PROBLEMS
CORONARY DISEASE
DISPROPORTION BETWEEN SUPPLY
(THRU CORONARIES) AND DEMAND

FLOW THROUGH TUBES VARIES WITH
THE FOURTH POWER OF THE DIAMETER.

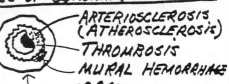

CAUSES OF CORONARY NARROWING.

  ARTERIOSCLEROSIS
(ATHEROSCLEROSIS)
THROMBOSIS
MURAL HEMORRHAGE
SPASM

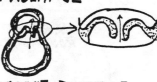

CORONARY HEART DISEASE

NARROWED
ROUGHENED
ARTERIES

MYOCARDIAL
ANOXIA ON
EXERTION
↓
PAIN IN
THE CHEST

ACUTE
MYOCARDIAL
ANOXIA
"HEART ATTACK"
↓
ARHYTHMIA ← INFARCT
(VENTRICULAR
FIBRILLATION)

COMPLICATIONS OF INFARCT

HEART FAILURE : ACUTE/CHRONIC
VALVE MALFUNCTION
RUPTURE
ARRHYTHMIA.

"CLOT BUSTERS" IN CORONARY THROMBOSIS

- USE WITH ASPIRIN
- FOLLOW WITH HEPARIN
- NOT HELPFUL AFTER 5 HOURS

DRUGS REDUCE MORTALITY AND
MYOCARDIAL DAMAGE
NO CLOT LYSIS TREATMENT MORTALITY
~11%
CLOT LYSIS MORTALITY ~ 8%
THREE MORE SURVIVALS / 100 PATIENTS
TREATED

AVAILABLE DRUGS
- TISSUE PLASMINOGEN ACTIVATOR (TPA)
- STREPTOKINASE
- MODIFIED LONG ACTING STREPTOKINASE

COMPLICATIONS
- STROKES
- ALLERGIC REACTIONS TO STREPTOKINASE

RESULTS
TPA MOST EFFECTIVE BUT MORE STROKES
1000 PATIENTS TREATED = 10 MORE
SURVIVORS - 1 MORE STROKE

THROMBOLYTIC THERAPY LESS
EFFECTIVE THAN IMMEDIATE
ANGIOPLASTY AND STENT

DIAGNOSIS AND TREATMENT

DIAGNOSIS
CLINICAL FEATURES
ELECTROCARDIOGRAM
(ARTERIOGRAM)

TREATMENT OF ACUTE EPISODE
UNBLOCK ARTERY IF POSSIBLE
CONSERVE AS MUCH HEART MUSCLE
AS POSSIBLE
MINIMIZE RISK OF COMPLICATIONS

MYOCARDIAL REVASCULARIZATION
"UNBLOCK" ARTERIES
REVASCULARIZE MUSCLE

LONG TERM MANAGEMENT : REDUCE RISK
FACTORS
CONTROL HYPERTENSION
LIPIDS
SMOKING
DIABETES

HYPERTENSIVE HEART DISEASE

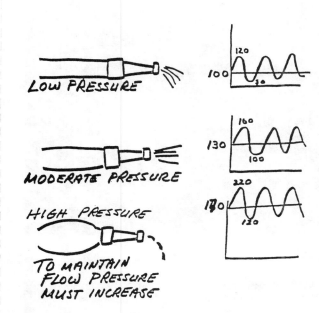

LOW PRESSURE

MODERATE PRESSURE

HIGH PRESSURE

TO MAINTAIN
FLOW PRESSURE
MUST INCREASE

ASPIRIN AND PLATELET FUNCTION

PLATELETS VERY SENSITIVE TO ASPIRIN (30MG/DAY)

ASPIRIN INACTIVATES (ACETYLATES) PLATELET
ENZYME REQUIRED FOR PLATELET AGGREGATION

ABILITY OF PLATELETS TO ADHERE TO ROUGH
SURFACE GREATLY REDUCED

EFFECT PERSISTS FOR ENTIRE 10 DAY LIFE
SPAN OF PLATELETS

ASPIRIN AND CARDIOVASCULAR DISEASE

A BABY ASPIRIN A DAY (80MG) PRODUCES
NON FUNCTIONAL PLATELETS.

IN SUSPECTED HEART ATTACK, ASPIRIN
RAPIDLY ABSORBED IN 20 MIN. AND
PLATELET FUNCTION EFFECTS IN AN HOUR

CARDIOVASCULAR DISEASE RISK FACTORS

HIGH CHOLESTEROL
HYPERTENSION
DIABETES
SMOKING
HIGH HOMOCYSTEINE

VALVULAR HEART DISEASE NOW AND INTO THE NEXT CENTURY

RHEUMATIC HEART DISEASE IS NOT
A PROBLEM IN DEVELOPED COUNTRIES

MAJOR VALVE LESIONS

- MITRAL VALVE PROLAPSE
- AORTIC STENOSIS RESULTING FROM
  BICUSPID AORTIC VALVE
  AGEING TRICUSPID AORTIC VALVE

DIAGNOSIS AND MANAGEMENT OF HEART MURMUR

- IS THERE A STRUCTURAL VALVE LESION?
- WHAT IS IT?
- WHAT ARE THE HEMODYNAMIC EFFECTS?
- SHOULD THE SUBJECT RECEIVE
  PROPHYLACTIC ANTIBIOTICS?

ROLE OF ULTRASOUND IN DIAGNOSIS AND MANAGEMENT

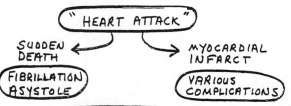

"HEART ATTACK"

SUDDEN DEATH → FIBRILLATION ASYSTOLE

MYOCARDIAL INFARCT → VARIOUS COMPLICATIONS

TREATMENT
RESTORE FLOW THROUGH BLOCKED ARTERY
- THROMBOLYTIC AGENTS
- IMMEDIATE ANGIOPLASTY

LONGER TERM MANAGEMENT OF SYMPTOMATIC
CORONARY HEART DISEASE

- ANGIOPLASTY
- CORONARY ARTERY BYPASS GRAFTS (CABG)
  ARTERIES FAVORED OVER
  VEINS FOR GRAFTING
- MIDCAB

REDUCE RISK OF CORONARY DISEASE

CONTROL RISK FACTORS
- SMOKING
- HYPERTENSION
- LIPIDS
- DIABETES

REDUCE RISK
- PRUDENT DIET
- WEIGHT CONTROL
- EXERCISE

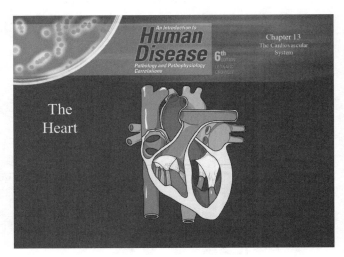

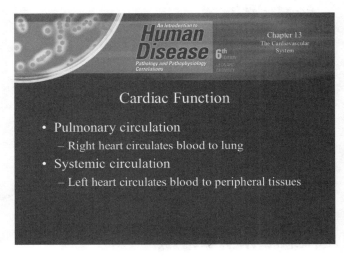

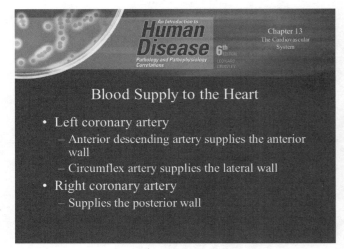

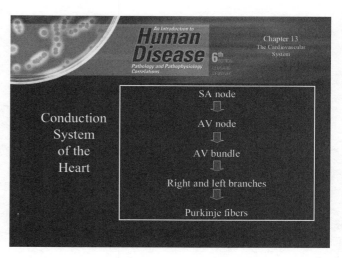

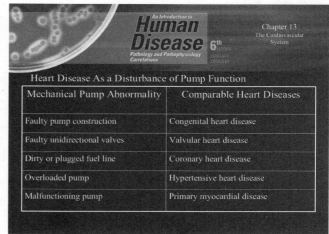

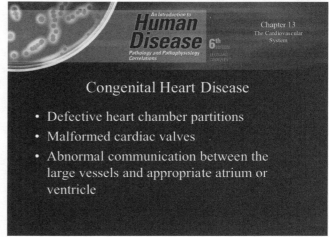

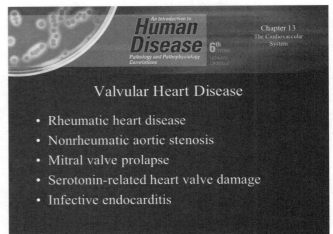

Valvular Heart Disease

- Rheumatic heart disease
- Nonrheumatic aortic stenosis
- Mitral valve prolapse
- Serotonin-related heart valve damage
- Infective endocarditis

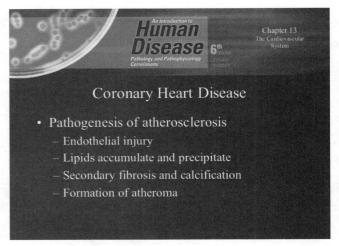

Coronary Heart Disease

- Pathogenesis of atherosclerosis
  - Endothelial injury
  - Lipids accumulate and precipitate
  - Secondary fibrosis and calcification
  - Formation of atheroma

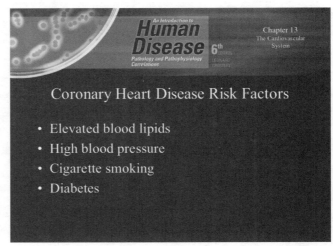

Coronary Heart Disease Risk Factors

- Elevated blood lipids
- High blood pressure
- Cigarette smoking
- Diabetes

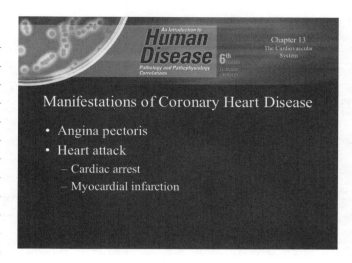

Manifestations of Coronary Heart Disease

- Angina pectoris
- Heart attack
  - Cardiac arrest
  - Myocardial infarction

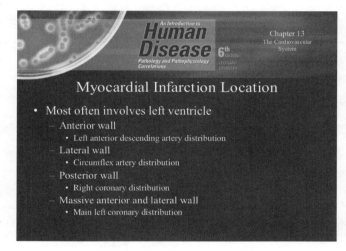

Myocardial Infarction Location

- Most often involves left ventricle
  - Anterior wall
    - Left anterior descending artery distribution
  - Lateral wall
    - Circumflex artery distribution
  - Posterior wall
    - Right coronary distribution
  - Massive anterior and lateral wall
    - Main left coronary distribution

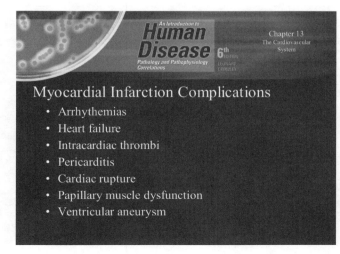

Myocardial Infarction Complications

- Arrhythemias
- Heart failure
- Intracardiac thrombi
- Pericarditis
- Cardiac rupture
- Papillary muscle dysfunction
- Ventricular aneurysm

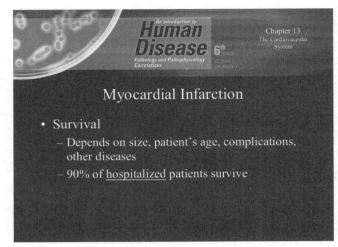

Myocardial Infarction

- Survival
  - Depends on size, patient's age, complications, other diseases
  - 90% of <u>hospitalized</u> patients survive

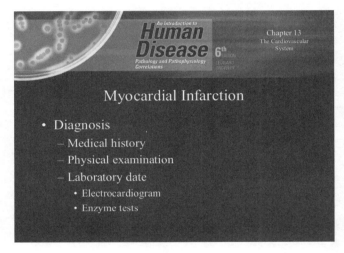

Myocardial Infarction

- Diagnosis
  - Medical history
  - Physical examination
  - Laboratory date
    - Electrocardiogram
    - Enzyme tests

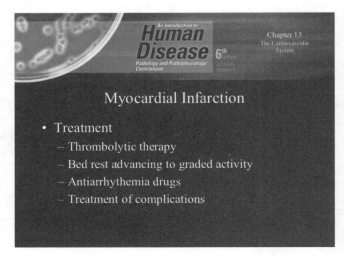

Myocardial Infarction

- Treatment
  - Thrombolytic therapy
  - Bed rest advancing to graded activity
  - Antiarrhythemia drugs
  - Treatment of complications

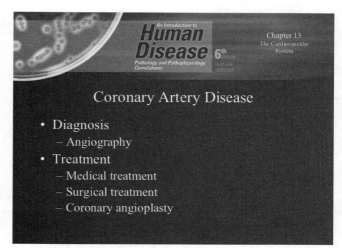

Coronary Artery Disease

- Diagnosis
  - Angiography
- Treatment
  - Medical treatment
  - Surgical treatment
  - Coronary angioplasty

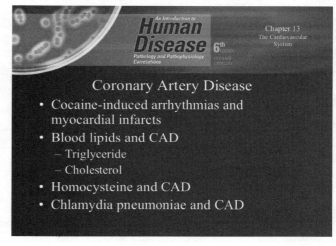

Coronary Artery Disease

- Cocaine-induced arrhythmias and myocardial infarcts
- Blood lipids and CAD
  - Triglyceride
  - Cholesterol
- Homocysteine and CAD
- Chlamydia pneumoniae and CAD

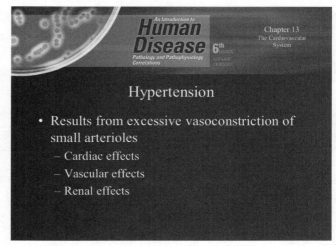

Hypertension

- Results from excessive vasoconstriction of small arterioles
  - Cardiac effects
  - Vascular effects
  - Renal effects

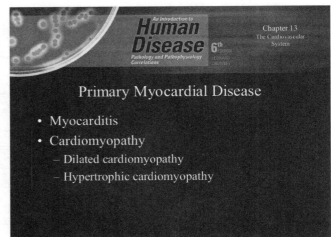

Primary Myocardial Disease

- Myocarditis
- Cardiomyopathy
  - Dilated cardiomyopathy
  - Hypertrophic cardiomyopathy

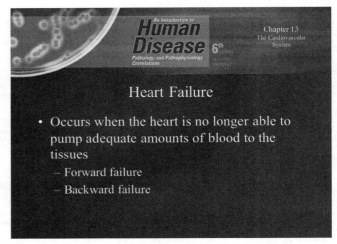

Heart Failure

- Occurs when the heart is no longer able to pump adequate amounts of blood to the tissues
  - Forward failure
  - Backward failure

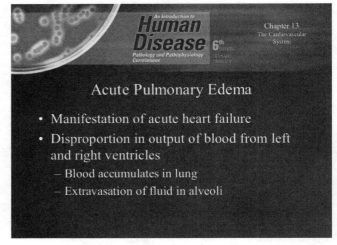

Acute Pulmonary Edema

- Manifestation of acute heart failure
- Disproportion in output of blood from left and right ventricles
  - Blood accumulates in lung
  - Extravasation of fluid in alveoli

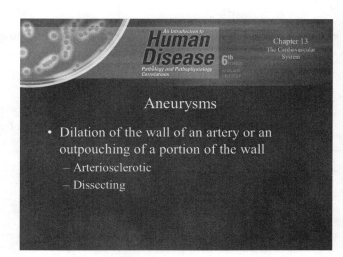

Aneurysms

- Dilation of the wall of an artery or an outpouching of a portion of the wall
  - Arteriosclerotic
  - Dissecting

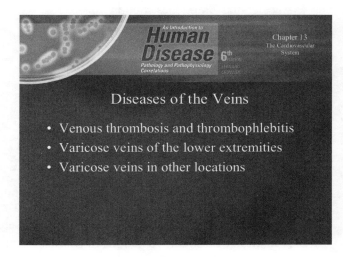

Diseases of the Veins

- Venous thrombosis and thrombophlebitis
- Varicose veins of the lower extremities
- Varicose veins in other locations

Chapter Outline

The chapter outline provides you with an organizational guide to the topics and ideas presented in this chapter of the text.

Study Questions

The following questions are provided as a test for comprehension and as a study guide for use with the text chapters. Additional study material is located at http://health.jbpub.com/humandisease/, which contains useful eLearning tools such as an A&P review, animated flashcards, interactive online glossary, crossword puzzles, and Web links.

Key Terms

Define the following terms:

1. Heme _____

2. Globin _____

3. Bilirubin _____

4. Anemia _____

5. Polycythemia _____

6. Hemochromatosis _____

Fill-in-the-Blank

1. The usual survival time of red cells in the circulation is _____.

2. The normal number of reticulocytes in the circulation is approximately _____ percent.

3. _____ is the usual cause of hypochromic, microcytic anemia in a middle-aged man.

4. Some patients have congenital deficiencies of the red cell enzymes that are required to metabolize glucose as a source of energy. These patients often have _____.

5. The disease in which there is an excess of iron in the body is called _____.

6. Infectious mononucleosis is caused by _____.

7. A young red cell is called a _____ and it survives in the circulation about _____ days. Worn-out red cells are destroyed primarily in _____. The hemoglobin is broken down and its components are recycled.

True/False

1. Tell whether each statement is true or false regarding iron deficiency anemia. If false, explain why the statement is incorrect.

   a. It may result from a bleeding ulcer. _____

   _____

   b. It may result from excessive blood donations. _____

   _____

   c. It may result from a deficiency of vitamins required for efficient blood production. _____

   _____

   d. It may result from excessive menstrual blood loss. _____

   _____

Identification

1. List the five white blood cells in the circulation and indicate their functions.

   a. _____

   b. _____

   c. _____

   d. _____

   e. _____

2. List three laboratory tests that are useful to measure iron stores, iron transport, and iron metabolism.

   a. _____

   b. _____

   c. _____

3. The macrocytic anemia resulting from inability to absorb vitamin B_{12} as a result of atrophy of gastric mucosa is called pernicious anemia. List three other causes of macrocytic anemia caused by inability to absorb or utilize vitamin B_{12}.

   a. _____

   b. _____

   c. _____

4. List four causes of hereditary hemolytic anemia.

   a. _____

   b. _____

   c. _____

   d. _____

5. List two treatments that are suitable for treating a patient with aplastic anemia.

   a. _____

   b. _____

6. List three diseases that are associated with secondary polycythemia.

   a. _____

   b. _____

   c. _____

Discussion Questions

1. Where does bilirubin come from? _____

   _____

   _____

   _____

2. Describe the uptake, transport, utilization, and storage of iron. (*Hint:* See Fig. 14-3.) _____

_____

_____

_____

3. What is the difference between the etiologic and the morphologic classifications of anemia? _____

_____

_____

_____

4. Outline a simple etiologic classification of anemia. _____

_____

_____

_____

5. What are the functions of the spleen? What happens if the spleen is removed? _____

_____

_____

_____

6. What are the clinical manifestations of infectious mononucleosis? How is the disease treated? _____

_____

_____

_____

7. How does primary polycythemia differ from secondary polycythemia? _____

_____

_____

_____

8. What is the difference between polycythemia and thrombocytopenia? _____

_____

_____

_____

9. What is the cause of aplastic anemia? How is it treated? _____

_____

_____

_____

10. What is the difference between aplastic anemia and hemolytic anemia? _____

_____

_____

_____

11. What is hemochromatosis? How is the condition diagnosed? How is it treated? _____

_____

_____

_____

12. What is the lymphatic system? How is it organized? What are the major cells in the lymphatic system? What are the major functions of the lymphatic system? _____

_____

_____

_____

13. List the morphologic features found in aplastic anemia (anemia due to bone marrow failure). _____

_____

_____

_____

14. What conditions are associated with megaloblastic anemia? _____

_____

_____

_____

THE "BONE MARROW FACTORY"

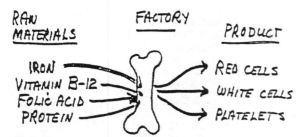

RAW MATERIALS | FACTORY | PRODUCT

IRON
VITAMIN B-12
FOLIC ACID
PROTEIN

→ RED CELLS
→ WHITE CELLS
→ PLATELETS

PRODUCTION AND DELIVERY MAY NOT CORRESPOND

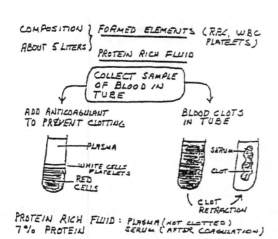

COMPOSITION } FORMED ELEMENTS (RBC, WBC
ABOUT 5 LITERS }   PLATELETS)
              PROTEIN RICH FLUID

COLLECT SAMPLE OF BLOOD IN TUBE

ADD ANTICOAGULANT TO PREVENT CLOTTING

BLOOD CLOTS IN TUBE

PLASMA
WHITE CELLS
PLATELETS
RED CELLS

SERUM
CLOT

CLOT RETRACTION

PROTEIN RICH FLUID : PLASMA (NOT CLOTTED)
7% PROTEIN   SERUM (AFTER COAGULATION)

ANEMIA

| INADEQUATE PRODUCTION | EXCESSIVE LOSS |

RAW MATERIAL DEFICIENCY
- IRON
- VITAMIN B-12
- FOLIC ACID

FACTORY INOPERATIVE
- DESTRUCTION
- REPLACEMENT

EXTERNAL LOSS

INTRAVASCULAR DESTRUCTION (HEMOLYTIC ANEMIA)
- HEREDITARY
- ACQUIRED

LIFE CYCLE OF THE RED CELL

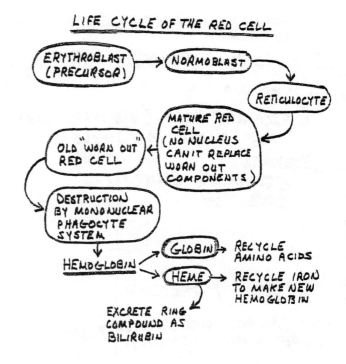

ERYTHROBLAST (PRECURSOR) → NORMOBLAST → RETICULOCYTE

MATURE RED CELL (NO NUCLEUS CAN'T REPLACE WORN OUT COMPONENTS)

OLD "WORN OUT" RED CELL

DESTRUCTION BY MONONUCLEAR PHAGOCYTE SYSTEM

HEMOGLOBIN → GLOBIN → RECYCLE AMINO ACIDS
          → HEME → RECYCLE IRON TO MAKE NEW HEMOGLOBIN

EXCRETE RING COMPOUND AS BILIRUBIN

CLASSIFICATION

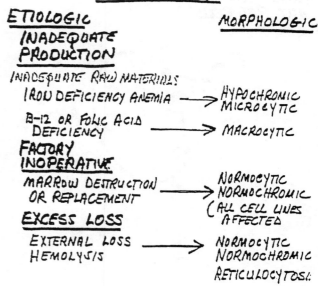

ETIOLOGIC | MORPHOLOGIC

INADEQUATE PRODUCTION

INADEQUATE RAW MATERIALS
IRON DEFICIENCY ANEMIA → HYPOCHROMIC MICROCYTIC

B-12 OR FOLIC ACID DEFICIENCY → MACROCYTIC

FACTORY INOPERATIVE
MARROW DESTRUCTION OR REPLACEMENT → NORMOCYTIC NORMOCHROMIC (ALL CELL LINES AFFECTED)

EXCESS LOSS
EXTERNAL LOSS HEMOLYSIS → NORMOCYTIC NORMOCHROMIC RETICULOCYTOSIS

IRON DEFICIENCY ANEMIA

A HYPOCHROMIC MICROCYTIC ANEMIA

1. INADEQUATE INTAKE

2. EXCESSIVE LOSS (VIA HgB LOSS AND FAILURE TO RECYCLE)

TREATMENT:
  ESTABLISH CAUSE!!!!
  GIVE IRON

IRON METABOLISM

IRON ABSORBED WITH DIFFICULTY AND EXCRETED WITH DIFFICULTY.

IRON INGESTED IN FOOD
IRON RECYCLED FROM WORN OUT RED CELLS
} IRON FOR HGB SYNTHESIS → RED CELLS

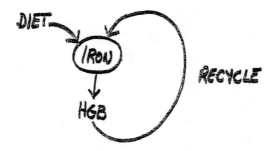

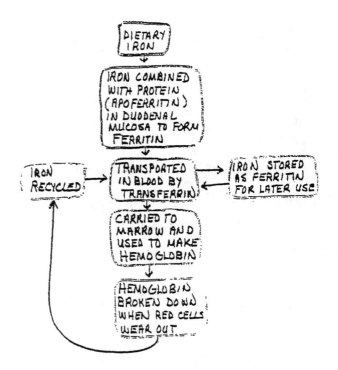

IRON DEFICIENCY AND EXCESS

TESTS TO MEASURE IRON STORAGE AND METABOLISM

FERRITIN IN SERUM: A MEASURE OF TOTAL IRON STORES

SERUM IRON AND IRON BINDING CAPACITY OF BLOOD TRANSPORT PROTEIN

PERCENT SATURATION OF IRON BINDING PROTEIN

IRON DEFICIENCY
  DIETARY
  CHRONIC BLOOD LOSS

IRON OVERLOAD : HEMOCHROMATOSIS
  AUTOSOMAL RECESSIVE DISEASE
  TISSUES OVERLOADED WITH IRON
  SECONDARY ORGAN DAMAGE
      CIRRHOSIS
      DIABETES
      IRON DEPOSITS IN SKIN DARKEN SKIN
      CARDIAC MUSCLE DAMAGE
  SCREENING FOR DISEASE RECOMMENDED
  TREATMENT BY PHLEBOTOMY

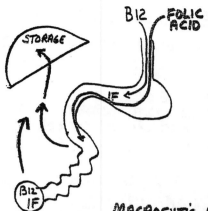

B12   FOLIC ACID

STORAGE

IF

B12 IF

DIAGNOSIS: MACROCYTIC ANEMIA
MEGALOBLASTIC MARROW
LOW B12 or FOLIC ACID

TREATMENT: CORRECT CAUSE
GIVE PARENTERAL B12
OR FOLIC ACID
(DEPENDING ON CAUSE)

B12 DEFICIENCY

B12 IN FOOD + GASTRIC DIGESTION + INTRINSIC FACTOR

→ B12·IF COMPLEX + ABSORPTION IN ILEUM → HEMATOPOIESIS

INADEQUATE B-12 INTAKE	DIETARY (RARE)
INADEQUATE GASTRIC DIGESTION	GASTRECTOMY "STOMACH STAPLING"
INTRINSIC FACTOR DEFICIENCY	PERNICIOUS ANEMIA
INTESTINAL MALABSORPTION	SMALL BOWEL DISEASE

ANEMIA CAUSED BY IMPAIRED MARROW FUNCTION

MILD: ANEMIA OF CHRONIC DISEASE

RELATED TO THE CHRONIC DISEASE AND IMPROVES WHEN THE DISEASE IMPROVES

USUALLY MILD TO MODERATE ANEMIA. WHITE CELLS AND PLATELETS NORMAL

LOW SERUM IRON AND LOW SERUM IRON BINDING CAPACITY

ADEQUATE IRON IN MARROW

SEVERE: APLASTIC ANEMIA

ANEMIA OF MARROW INFILTRATION

A NORMOCYTIC ANEMIA
- LEUKEMIA
- METASTATIC CANCER
- OTHER CAUSES

DIAGNOSIS: BONE MARROW BIOPSY

TREATMENT: OF PRIMARY DISEASE

POLYCYTHEMIA

PRIMARY (POLYCYTHEMIA VERA)

SECONDARY (SYMPTOMATIC)
- CHRONIC LUNG DISEASE
- CONGENITAL HEART DISEASE (CYANOTIC)

MARROW DAMAGE ("APLASTIC ANEMIA")

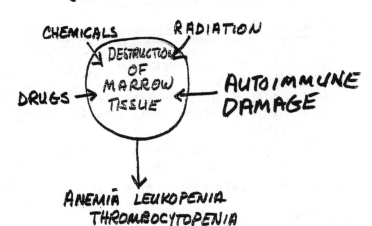

CHEMICALS · RADIATION

DRUGS → DESTRUCTION OF MARROW TISSUE ← AUTOIMMUNE DAMAGE

ANEMIA LEUKOPENIA
THROMBOCYTOPENIA

TREATMENT:
  SUPPORTIVE
  MARROW TRANSPLANT

ANEMIA OF BLOOD LOSS

- EXTERNAL BLOOD LOSS

- EXCESSIVE DESTRUCTION

  DEFECTIVE CELL
    - ABNORMAL SHAPE
    - ABNORMAL HEMOGLOBIN
    - ABNORMAL METABOLISM

  HOSTILE ENVIRONMENT
    - AUTOANTIBODIES
    - MECHANICAL TRAUMA

EVALUATION OF ANEMIA

- HISTORY

- PHYSICAL EXAMINATION

- EVALUATION OF "DELIVERY" OF CELLS
    BLOOD COUNT
    EXAMINE BLOOD SMEAR
    RETICULOCYTES / PLATELETS

- EVALUATION OF "PRODUCTION"

- SPECIAL STUDIES WHERE INDICATED

LEUKEMIA

CLASSIFICATION

BY CELL TYPE — GRANULOCYTE, MONOCYTE, LYMPHOCYTE

BY MATURITY OF CELL
- ACUTE = IMMATURE
- CHRONIC = MATURE

MANIFESTATIONS

1. FROM IMPAIRED MARROW FUNCTION
   - ANEMIA
   - THROMBOCYTOPENIA
   - REDUCED FUNCTIONALLY NORMAL WHITE CELLS
2. FROM INFILTRATION OF VISCERA
   - SPLENOMEGALY
   - HEPATOMEGALY
   - ENLARGED LYMPH NODES

MYELODYSPLASTIC SYNDROMES "PRELEUKEMIA"

MYELOMA : PLASMA CELL NEOPLASM

1. NODULAR (AND DIFFUSE) MARROW INFILTRATION

2. BONE DESTRUCTION

3. ELABORATION OF PROTEIN (HOMOGENEOUS = MONOCLONAL BAND)

PLASMA CELLS USUALLY REMAIN IN MARROW — PERIPHERAL BLOOD PLASMACYTOSIS DOES NOT OCCUR IN MOST CASES.

Notes

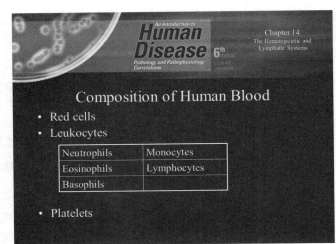

Composition of Human Blood

- Red cells
- Leukocytes

Neutrophils	Monocytes
Eosinophils	Lymphocytes
Basophils	

- Platelets

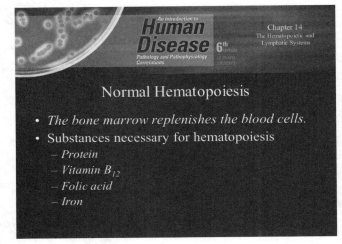

Normal Hematopoiesis

- *The bone marrow replenishes the blood cells.*
- Substances necessary for hematopoiesis
  - *Protein*
  - *Vitamin B_{12}*
  - *Folic acid*
  - *Iron*

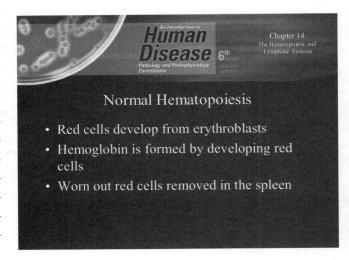

Normal Hematopoiesis

- Red cells develop from erythroblasts
- Hemoglobin is formed by developing red cells
- Worn out red cells removed in the spleen

Notes

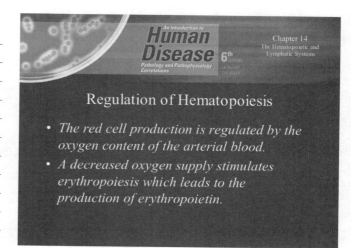

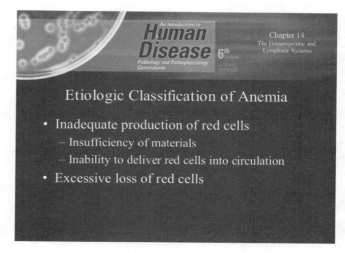

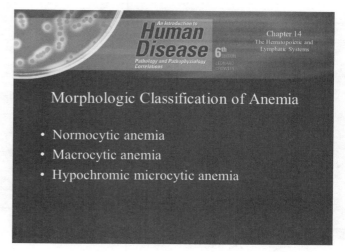

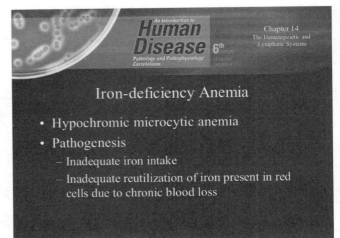

Iron-deficiency Anemia

- Hypochromic microcytic anemia
- Pathogenesis
  - Inadequate iron intake
  - Inadequate reutilization of iron present in red cells due to chronic blood loss

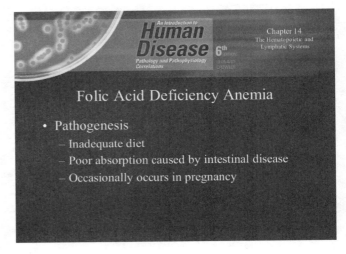

Folic Acid Deficiency Anemia

- Pathogenesis
  - Inadequate diet
  - Poor absorption caused by intestinal disease
  - Occasionally occurs in pregnancy

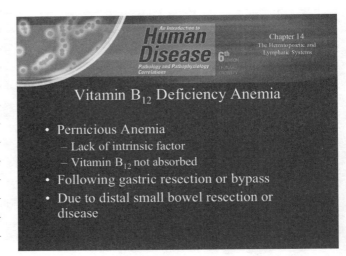

Vitamin B_{12} Deficiency Anemia

- Pernicious Anemia
  - Lack of intrinsic factor
  - Vitamin B_{12} not absorbed
- Following gastric resection or bypass
- Due to distal small bowel resection or disease

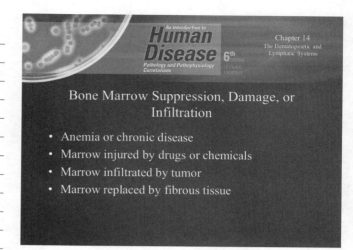

Bone Marrow Suppression, Damage, or Infiltration

- Anemia or chronic disease
- Marrow injured by drugs or chemicals
- Marrow infiltrated by tumor
- Marrow replaced by fibrous tissue

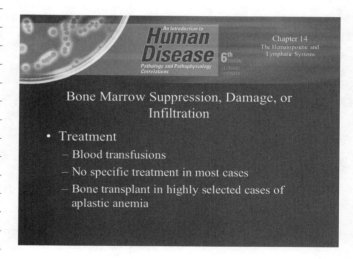

Bone Marrow Suppression, Damage, or Infiltration

- Treatment
  - Blood transfusions
  - No specific treatment in most cases
  - Bone transplant in highly selected cases of aplastic anemia

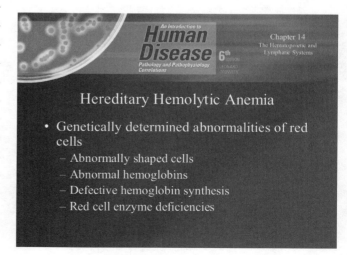

Hereditary Hemolytic Anemia

- Genetically determined abnormalities of red cells
  - Abnormally shaped cells
  - Abnormal hemoglobins
  - Defective hemoglobin synthesis
  - Red cell enzyme deficiencies

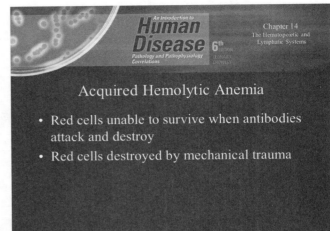

Acquired Hemolytic Anemia

- Red cells unable to survive when antibodies attack and destroy
- Red cells destroyed by mechanical trauma

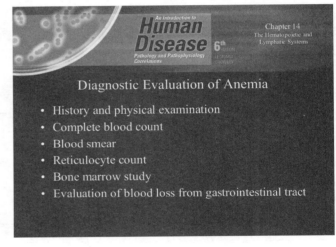

Diagnostic Evaluation of Anemia

- History and physical examination
- Complete blood count
- Blood smear
- Reticulocyte count
- Bone marrow study
- Evaluation of blood loss from gastrointestinal tract

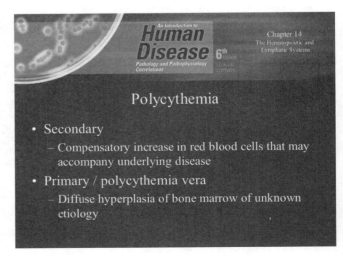

Polycythemia

- Secondary
  - Compensatory increase in red blood cells that may accompany underlying disease
- Primary / polycythemia vera
  - Diffuse hyperplasia of bone marrow of unknown etiology

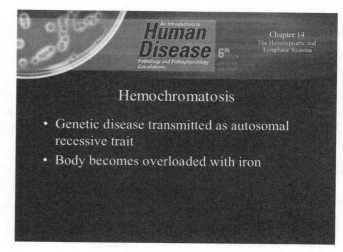

Hemochromatosis

- Genetic disease transmitted as autosomal recessive trait
- Body becomes overloaded with iron

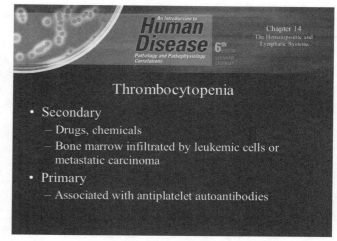

Thrombocytopenia

- Secondary
  - Drugs, chemicals
  - Bone marrow infiltrated by leukemic cells or metastatic carcinoma
- Primary
  - Associated with antiplatelet autoantibodies

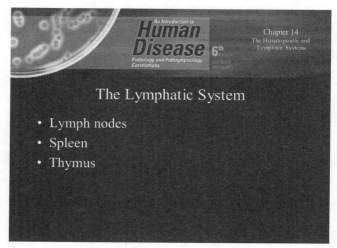

The Lymphatic System

- Lymph nodes
- Spleen
- Thymus

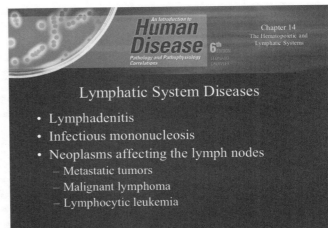

Lymphatic System Diseases

- Lymphadenitis
- Infectious mononucleosis
- Neoplasms affecting the lymph nodes
  - Metastatic tumors
  - Malignant lymphoma
  - Lymphocytic leukemia

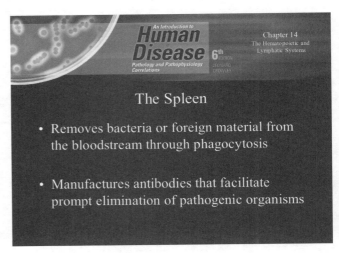

The Spleen

- Removes bacteria or foreign material from the bloodstream through phagocytosis

- Manufactures antibodies that facilitate prompt elimination of pathogenic organisms

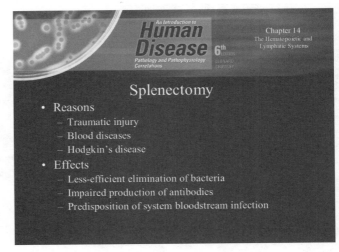

Splenectomy

- Reasons
  - Traumatic injury
  - Blood diseases
  - Hodgkin's disease
- Effects
  - Less-efficient elimination of bacteria
  - Impaired production of antibodies
  - Predisposition of system bloodstream infection

Chapter Outline

The chapter outline provides you with an organizational guide to the topics and ideas presented in this chapter of the text.

Oxygen Delivery: A Cooperative Effort
Structure and Function of the Lungs
    Bronchi, Bronchioles, and Alveoli
    Ventilation
    Gas Exchange
    Pulmonary Function Tests
    The Pleural Cavity
Pneumothorax
Atelectasis
    Obstructive Atelectasis
    Compression Atelectasis
Pneumonia
    Classification of Pneumonia
    Clinical Features of Pneumonia
    Severe Acute Respiratory Syndrome (SARS)
    Pneumocystis Pneumonia
Tuberculosis
    Course of a Tuberculous Infection
    Miliary Tuberculosis and Tuberculous Pneumonia
    Extrapulmonary Tuberculosis
    Diagnosis and Treatment of Tuberculosis
Bronchitis and Bronchiectasis
Chronic Obstructive Lung Disease
    Derangements of Pulmonary Structure and Function
    Pathogenesis of Emphysema
    Prevention and Treatment of Emphysema
    Emphysema as a Result of Alpha-1 Antitrypsin Deficiency
Bronchial Asthma
Respiratory Distress Syndrome
    Respiratory Distress Syndrome of Newborn Infants
    Adult Respiratory Distress Syndrome
Pulmonary Fibrosis
Lung Carcinoma

Study Questions

The following questions are provided as a test for comprehension and as a study guide for use with the text chapters. Additional study material is located at http://health.jbpub.com/humandisease/, which contains useful eLearning tools such as an A&P review, animated flashcards, interactive online glossary, crossword puzzles, and Web links.

Key Terms

Define the following terms:

1. Miliary tuberculosis _____

2. Pulmonary fibrosis _____

3. Pneumothorax _____

4. Pulmonary emphysema _____

5. Pneumonia _____

Fill-in-the-Blank

1. Movement of air in and out of the lungs is called _____, and movement of oxygen and carbon dioxide between alveoli and pulmonary capillaries is called _____.

2. Escape of air from the lung associated with collapse of the lung is called a _____.

3. Development of a positive (higher-than-atmospheric) pressure in the pleural cavity associated with collapse of the lung is called a _____, and this condition is treated by _____.

4. Collapse of part of the lung caused by obstruction of bronchi or bronchioles with absorption of the trapped air into the bloodstream is called _____.

5. The agent that causes severe acute respiratory syndrome (SARS) is _____.

6. Primary atypical pneumonia is caused by _____.

7. The characteristic multinucleated cell associated with the necrosis in tuberculosis is called a _____.

8. The skin test that detects hypersensitivity to the antigens in the tubercle bacillus as an indication of previous exposure to the organism is called the _____ test.

9. Deficiency of surfactant in the lungs of premature infants leads to a condition called _____.

10. The condition characterized by breathing difficulty caused by bronchospasm is called _____.

11. Progressive pulmonary fibrosis caused by inhalation of rock dust is called _____.

12. Pulmonary fibrosis caused by inhalation of asbestos fibers is called _____.

13. The disease caused by exposure to asbestos fibers may predispose a person to development of malignant lung and pleural tumors. The lung tumor is called a _____, and the pleural tumor is called a _____.

14. The disease characterized by chronic bronchitis associated with breakdown of alveolar septa, formation of cystic spaces throughout the lung, and loss of lung elasticity is called _____.

15. The incidence of pulmonary emphysema is _____.

16. _____ is the major factor responsible for the rising incidence of lung carcinoma in women.

17. _____ is a condition characterized by chronic inflammation with dilation of bronchi.

18. Inhalation of a foreign body in the lung may cause _____.

True/False

1. Tell whether each statement is true or false regarding the severe acute respiratory syndrome (SARS). If false, explain why the statement is incorrect.

   a. This highly communicable disease is caused by an unusual coronavirus. _____

   _____

   b. The virus can be transmitted by coughing and sneezing, and by the virus-contaminated hands of an infected patient.

   _____

   c. The virus responds to antiviral antibiotics. _____

   _____

   d. The lungs of severely affected SARS patients develop features characteristic of adult respiratory distress syndrome.

   _____

2. Tell whether each statement is true or false regarding the treatment of emphysema by lung volume reduction surgery (LVRS). If false, explain why the statement is incorrect.

   a. LVRS may be suitable for some patients who have emphysema restricted to the upper lobes of the lungs.

   _____

   b. LVRS involves resecting segments of emphysematous upper lobes in an effort to reduce the size of the overinflated lungs so that the less severely affected lower lobes can function more efficiently. _____

   _____

   c. The mortality rate for medically treated patients with emphysema is similar to the mortality rate for surgically treated patients. _____

   _____

   d. Surgical treatment is much more effective than medical treatment in almost all emphysema patients. _____

   _____

Identification

1. List three conditions that appear to be related to cigarette smoking.

   a. _____

   b. _____

   c. _____

Discussion Questions

1. How do the lungs function? _____
   _____
   _____
   _____

2. What is the difference between ventilation and gas exchange? _____
   _____
   _____
   _____

3. How is pulmonary function disturbed if the alveolar septa are thickened and scarred? _____
   _____
   _____
   _____

4. How is pneumonia classified? What are its major clinical features? _____
   _____
   _____
   _____

5. How does the tubercle bacillus differ in its staining reaction from other bacteria? _____
   _____
   _____
   _____

6. What factors determine the outcome of a tuberculous infection? _____
   _____
   _____
   _____

7. How does a cavity develop in lungs infected with tuberculosis? Is a person with a tuberculous cavity infectious to
   other people? _____
   _____
   _____
   _____

8. What type of inflammation is caused by the tubercle bacillus? _____
   _____
   _____
   _____

9. A patient has tuberculosis of the kidney, but no evidence of pulmonary tuberculosis is detected by means of a chest X-ray. How did this happen? _____

_____

_____

_____

10. What is meant by the term "inactive tuberculosis"? Under what circumstances may an old, inactive tuberculous infection become activated? What types of patients are susceptible to reactivation of a tuberculous infection?

_____

_____

_____

11. How does a pneumothorax occur? What is its effect on pulmonary function? _____

_____

_____

_____

12. What factors predispose a person to the development of pulmonary emphysema? How may it be prevented?

_____

_____

_____

13. A 35-year-old man has a pulmonary infiltrate with chills, fever, chest pain, and purulent sputum. What is the most likely diagnosis? _____

_____

_____

_____

14. A postoperative patient with a normal temperature has a pulmonary infiltrate, chest pain, and bloody sputum. What is the most likely diagnosis? _____

_____

_____

_____

15. What is the cause of interstitial pneumonia (primary atypical pneumonia)? _____

_____

_____

_____

RESPIRATORY SYSTEM

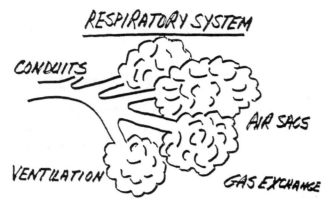

CONDUITS

AIR SACS

VENTILATION

GAS EXCHANGE

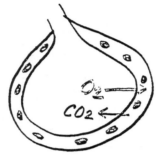

O_2

CO_2

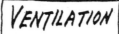

VENTILATION	GAS EXCHANGE
OPEN AIR PASSAGES	NORMAL ALVEOLI
NORMAL MOVEMENT OF DIAPHRAGM AND RIB CAGE	NORMAL PULMONARY BLOOD FLOW
NORMAL NEURO-MUSCULAR SYSTEM	

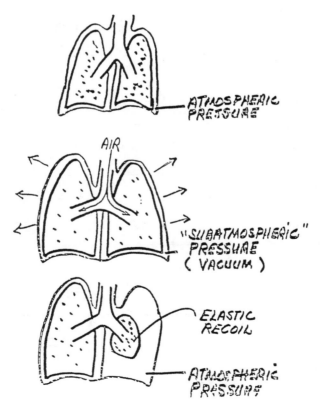

ATMOSPHERIC PRESSURE

AIR

"SUBATMOSPHERIC" PRESSURE (VACUUM)

ELASTIC RECOIL

ATMOSPHERIC PRESSURE

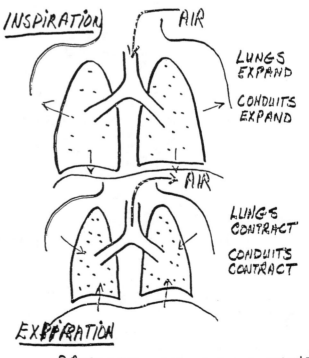

INSPIRATION   AIR

LUNGS EXPAND

CONDUITS EXPAND

AIR

LUNGS CONTRACT

CONDUITS CONTRACT

EXPIRATION

PRESSURE GRADIENTS MAINTAINED

PNEUMONIA

CLINICAL FEATURES

1. OF INFECTION
2. OF BRONCHIAL IRRITATION
3. OF PLEURAL IRRITATION
4. OF LOSS OF PULMONARY FUNCTION

TUBERCULOSIS

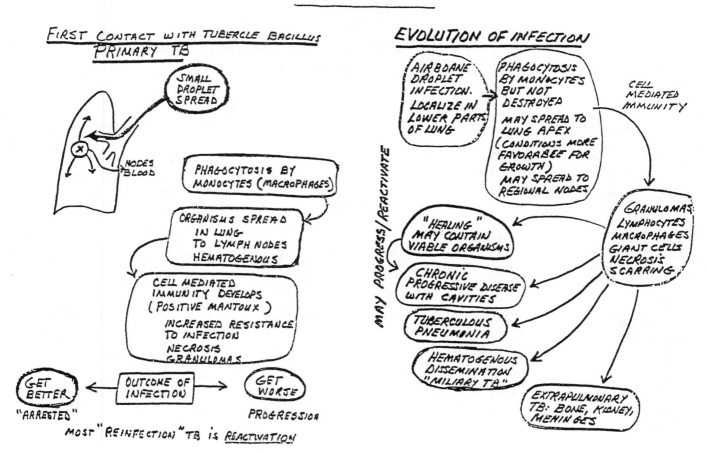

FIRST CONTACT WITH TUBERCLE BACILLUS
__PRIMARY TB__

SMALL DROPLET SPREAD

NODES BLOOD

PHAGOCYTOSIS BY MONOCYTES (MACROPHAGES)

ORGANISMS SPREAD IN LUNG TO LYMPH NODES HEMATOGENOUS

CELL MEDIATED IMMUNITY DEVELOPS (POSITIVE MANTOUX)
INCREASED RESISTANCE TO INFECTION NECROSIS GRANULOMAS

GET BETTER "ARRESTED" ← OUTCOME OF INFECTION → GET WORSE PROGRESSION

MOST "REINFECTION" TB is __REACTIVATION__

EVOLUTION OF INFECTION

AIRBORNE DROPLET INFECTION. LOCALIZE IN LOWER PARTS OF LUNG

PHAGOCYTOSIS BY MONOCYTES BUT NOT DESTROYED
MAY SPREAD TO LUNG APEX (CONDITIONS MORE FAVORABLE FOR GROWTH)
MAY SPREAD TO REGIONAL NODES

CELL MEDIATED IMMUNITY

MAY PROGRESS/REACTIVATE

"HEALING" MAY CONTAIN VIABLE ORGANISMS

CHRONIC PROGRESSIVE DISEASE WITH CAVITIES

TUBERCULOUS PNEUMONIA

HEMATOGENOUS DISSEMINATION "MILIARY TB"

GRANULOMAS LYMPHOCYTES MACROPHAGES GIANT CELLS NECROSIS SCARRING

EXTRAPULMONARY TB: BONE, KIDNEY, MENINGES

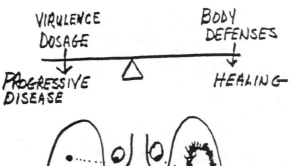

VIRULENCE
DOSAGE

BODY
DEFENSES

PROGRESSIVE
DISEASE

HEALING

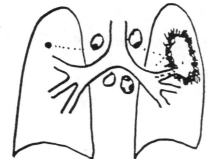

PRIMARY TB
"REINFECTION" (REACTIVATION) TB
TB AND IMPAIRED IMMUNE DEFENSES
ANTIBIOTIC RESISTANT TB

EMPHYSEMA

RUPTURE OF
ALVEOLAR SEPTA

REDUCTION
OF PULMONARY
VASCULAR BED

LOSS OF
LUNG
ELASTICITY

INADEQUATE
GAS EXCHANGE

COMPRESSION
OF ALVEOLI
AND BRONCHIOLES

INADEQUATE
OXYGENATION
AND CO_2
ELIMINATION

TRAPPING OF
AIR IN LUNGS

INADEQUATE
INEFFICIENT
LUNG FUNCTION

PATHOGENESIS

CHRONIC
BRONCHITIS

INCREASED
SECRETIONS

POOR
DRAINAGE

INFECTIONS

COUGH

ALVEOLAR
DAMAGE

[ENZYME DEFICIENCY]

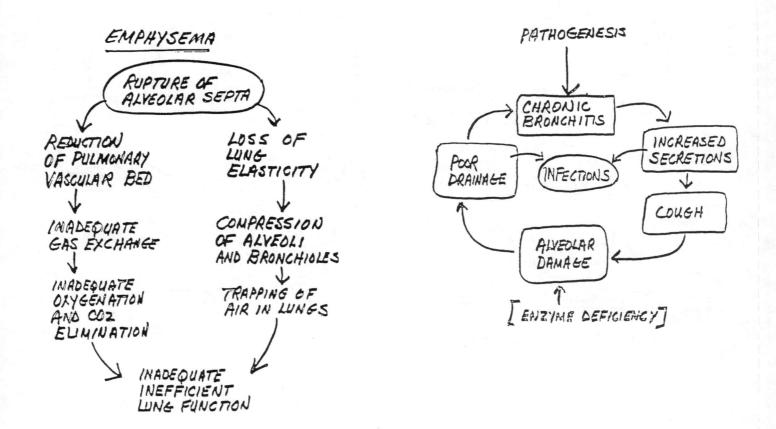

SMOKING AND LUNG DISEASE

EMPHYSEMA   LUNG CANCER

EVIDENCE -
- EPIDEMIOLOGIC
- EXPERIMENTAL

LUNG CANCER MORTALITY
IN WOMEN NOW EXCEEDS
BREAST CARCINOMA
MORTALITY!

RESPIRATORY DISTRESS SYNDROMES

NEONATAL
"PREMIES"
C SECTIONS
DIABETIC MOTHER
↓
INADEQUATE
SURFACTANT
↓
POOR ALVEOLAR
EXPANSION·COLLAPSE
INCREASED CAPILLARY
PERMEABILITY
↓
PROTEIN RICH FLUID
LEAKS

Rx MATERNAL
CORTICOSTEROIDS

ADULT
DIRECT LUNG DAMAGE
- LUNG TRAUMA
- ASPIRATION
- IRRITANT - TOXIC GA.
INDIRECT LUNG DAMAGE
- POOR PERFUSION
  (TRAUMA - SEPSIS)
↓
INCREASED CAPILLARY
PERMEABILITY
REDUCED SURFACTANT
↓
PROTEIN RICH FLUID
LEAKS

SUPPORTIVE
POS. PRESSURE O2

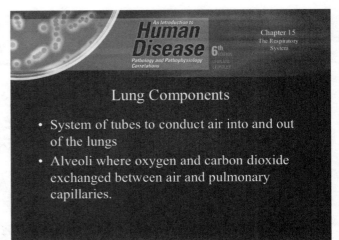

Lung Components

- System of tubes to conduct air into and out of the lungs
- Alveoli where oxygen and carbon dioxide exchanged between air and pulmonary capillaries.

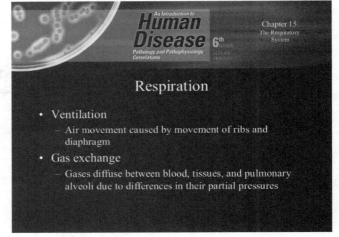

Respiration

- Ventilation
  - Air movement caused by movement of ribs and diaphragm
- Gas exchange
  - Gases diffuse between blood, tissues, and pulmonary alveoli due to differences in their partial pressures

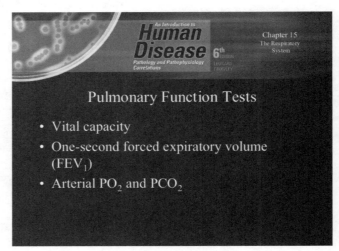

Pulmonary Function Tests

- Vital capacity
- One-second forced expiratory volume (FEV_1)
- Arterial PO_2 and PCO_2

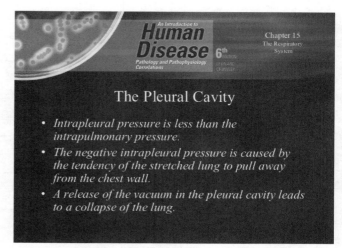

The Pleural Cavity

- *Intrapleural pressure is less than the intrapulmonary pressure.*
- *The negative intrapleural pressure is caused by the tendency of the stretched lung to pull away from the chest wall.*
- *A release of the vacuum in the pleural cavity leads to a collapse of the lung.*

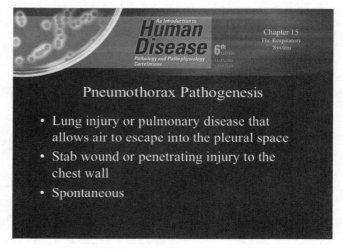

Pneumothorax Pathogenesis

- Lung injury or pulmonary disease that allows air to escape into the pleural space
- Stab wound or penetrating injury to the chest wall
- Spontaneous

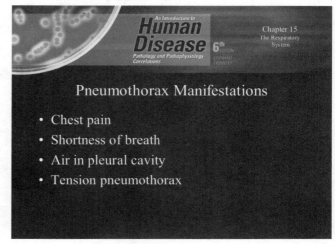

Pneumothorax Manifestations

- Chest pain
- Shortness of breath
- Air in pleural cavity
- Tension pneumothorax

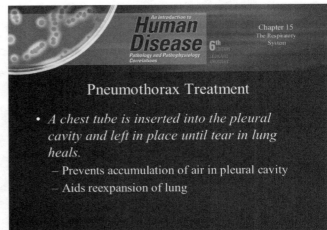

Pneumothorax Treatment

- *A chest tube is inserted into the pleural cavity and left in place until tear in lung heals.*
  - Prevents accumulation of air in pleural cavity
  - Aids reexpansion of lung

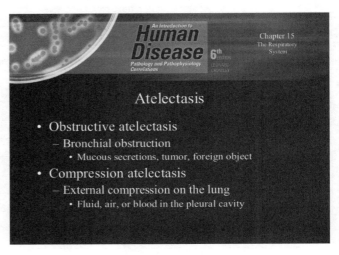

Atelectasis

- Obstructive atelectasis
  - Bronchial obstruction
    - Mucous secretions, tumor, foreign object
- Compression atelectasis
  - External compression on the lung
    - Fluid, air, or blood in the pleural cavity

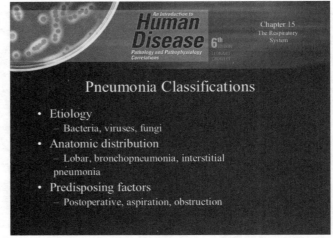

Pneumonia Classifications

- Etiology
  - Bacteria, viruses, fungi
- Anatomic distribution
  - Lobar, bronchopneumonia, interstitial pneumonia
- Predisposing factors
  - Postoperative, aspiration, obstruction

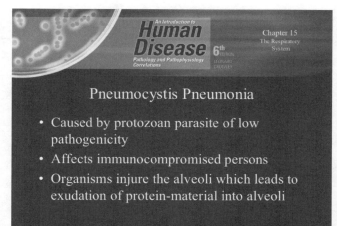

Pneumocystis Pneumonia

- Caused by protozoan parasite of low pathogenicity
- Affects immunocompromised persons
- Organisms injure the alveoli which leads to exudation of protein-material into alveoli

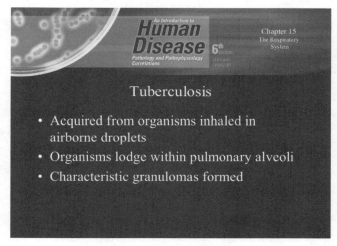

Tuberculosis

- Acquired from organisms inhaled in airborne droplets
- Organisms lodge within pulmonary alveoli
- Characteristic granulomas formed

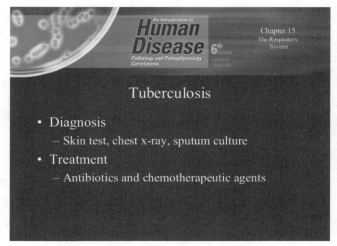

Tuberculosis

- Diagnosis
  - Skin test, chest x-ray, sputum culture
- Treatment
  - Antibiotics and chemotherapeutic agents

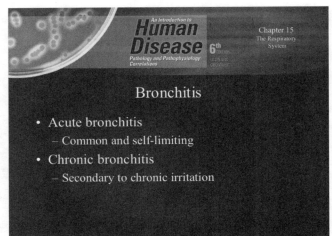

Bronchitis

- Acute bronchitis
  - Common and self-limiting
- Chronic bronchitis
  - Secondary to chronic irritation

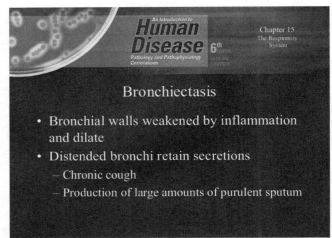

Bronchiectasis

- Bronchial walls weakened by inflammation and dilate
- Distended bronchi retain secretions
  - Chronic cough
  - Production of large amounts of purulent sputum

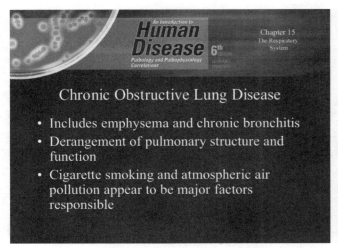

Chronic Obstructive Lung Disease

- Includes emphysema and chronic bronchitis
- Derangement of pulmonary structure and function
- Cigarette smoking and atmospheric air pollution appear to be major factors responsible

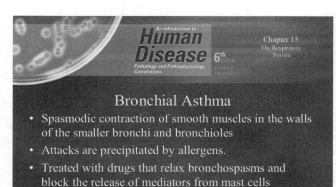

Bronchial Asthma

- Spasmodic contraction of smooth muscles in the walls of the smaller bronchi and bronchioles
- Attacks are precipitated by allergens.
- Treated with drugs that relax bronchospasms and block the release of mediators from mast cells

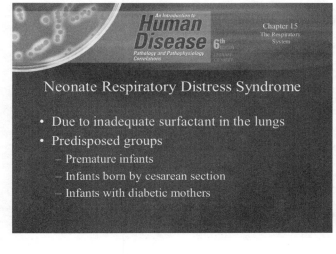

Neonate Respiratory Distress Syndrome

- Due to inadequate surfactant in the lungs
- Predisposed groups
  - Premature infants
  - Infants born by cesarean section
  - Infants with diabetic mothers

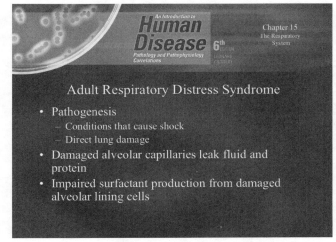

Adult Respiratory Distress Syndrome

- Pathogenesis
  - Conditions that cause shock
  - Direct lung damage
- Damaged alveolar capillaries leak fluid and protein
- Impaired surfactant production from damaged alveolar lining cells

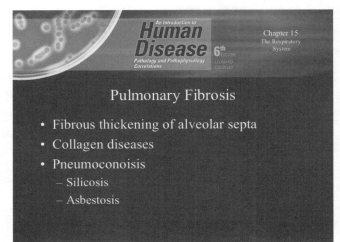

Pulmonary Fibrosis

- Fibrous thickening of alveolar septa
- Collagen diseases
- Pneumoconoisis
  - Silicosis
  - Asbestosis

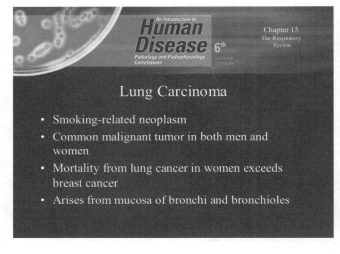

Lung Carcinoma

- Smoking-related neoplasm
- Common malignant tumor in both men and women
- Mortality from lung cancer in women exceeds breast cancer
- Arises from mucosa of bronchi and bronchioles

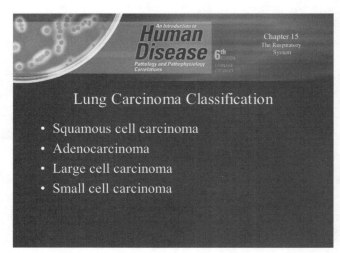

Lung Carcinoma Classification

- Squamous cell carcinoma
- Adenocarcinoma
- Large cell carcinoma
- Small cell carcinoma

Chapter Outline

The chapter outline provides you with an organizational guide to the topics and ideas presented in this chapter of the text.

Study Questions

The following questions are provided as a test for comprehension and as a study guide for use with the text chapters. Additional study material is located at http://health.jbpub.com/humandisease/, which contains useful eLearning tools such as an A&P review, animated flashcards, interactive online glossary, crossword puzzles, and Web links.

Key Terms

Define the following terms:

1. Mammogram _____

2. Gynecomastia _____

3. Axilla _____

4. Estrogen _____

5. Progestin _____

6. Mastectomy _____

7. Tamoxifen _____

8. Adjuvant chemotherapy _____

Fill-in-the-Blank

1. Persons with mutations of the tumor suppressor genes BRCA1 or BRCA2 have a greatly increased risk of not only breast carcinoma but also _____ carcinoma.

2. A well-circumscribed benign tumor occurring in the breast of a young woman is called a _____.

3. Breast enlargement in the male breast is called _____.

4. Following treatment of an invasive breast carcinoma, most patients are also treated with drugs or hormones. This type of treatment is called _____.

5. When examining axillary lymph nodes from patients with breast carcinoma, it is possible to identify and examine the first lymph node that receives lymphatic drainage from the axilla. This node is called a _____.

True/False

Tell whether each statement is true or false. If false, explain why the statement is incorrect.

1. A mutation of either the BRCA1 or BRCA2 gene increases the long-term risk of both breast and ovarian carcinoma.

   _____

2. Long-term treatment of postmenopausal patients with estrogen and progestin increases the risk of breast carcinoma.

   _____

3. When treating breast carcinoma, the long-term results of total mastectomy with axillary lymph node dissection are much better than the results of segmental mastectomy or lumpectomy followed by radiation therapy. _____

   _____

4. An estrogen receptor-positive breast carcinoma has a better prognosis than a breast carcinoma lacking hormone receptors. _____

_____

5. The prognosis of a breast carcinoma in which the HER-2 gene is amplified is much better than that of a breast carcinoma lacking an amplified HER-2 gene. _____

_____

6. An axillary lymph node containing metastatic carcinoma is called a sentinal lymph node. _____

_____

7. An estrogen receptor-negative breast carcinoma is usually treated with the drug tamoxifen. _____

_____

8. Adjuvant therapy for most patients with breast carcinoma usually consists of hormonal therapy and/or chemotherapy.

_____

Identify

1. What are the three common conditions that cause a lump in the breast?

a. _____

b. _____

c. _____

2. Which three laboratory tests are performed on breast carcinoma tissue to assess prognosis and guide treatment?

a. _____

b. _____

c. _____

Discussion Questions

1. Describe the methods used to treat breast carcinoma surgically. _____

_____

_____

_____

2. How can benign breast conditions be distinguished from breast cancer? _____

_____

_____

_____

3. What are the applications and limitations of a mammogram? _____
_____
_____
_____

4. What factors predispose a person to breast carcinoma? _____
_____
_____
_____

5. What is the role of heredity in regard to breast carcinoma? _____
_____
_____
_____

6. A 67-year-old woman has a lump in the breast. Which diagnostic procedures will assist the physician in determining the nature of the lump? _____
_____
_____
_____

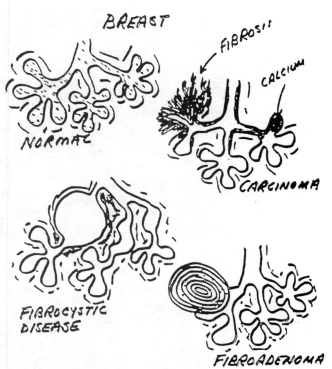

PATHOGENESIS
EVOLUTION OF BREAST CARCINOMA
CONCEPT OF INSITU AND INVASIVE CARCINOMA
HEREDITY AND BREAST CARCINOMA
HORMONES AND BREAST CARCINOMA

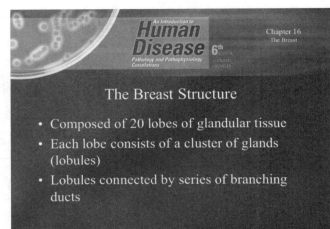

The Breast Structure

- Composed of 20 lobes of glandular tissue
- Each lobe consists of a cluster of glands (lobules)
- Lobules connected by series of branching ducts

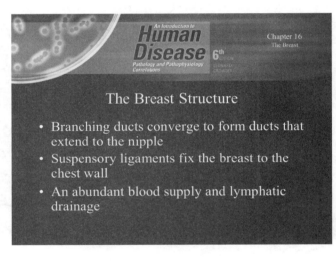

The Breast Structure

- Branching ducts converge to form ducts that extend to the nipple
- Suspensory ligaments fix the breast to the chest wall
- An abundant blood supply and lymphatic drainage

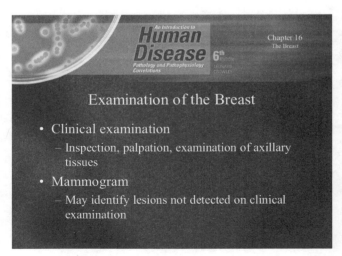

Examination of the Breast

- Clinical examination
  - Inspection, palpation, examination of axillary tissues
- Mammogram
  - May identify lesions not detected on clinical examination

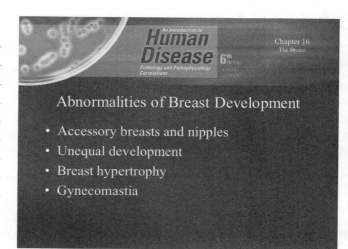

Abnormalities of Breast Development

- Accessory breasts and nipples
- Unequal development
- Breast hypertrophy
- Gynecomastia

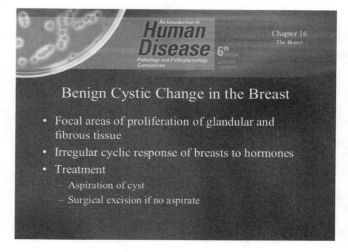

Benign Cystic Change in the Breast

- Focal areas of proliferation of glandular and fibrous tissue
- Irregular cyclic response of breasts to hormones
- Treatment
  - Aspiration of cyst
  - Surgical excision if no aspirate

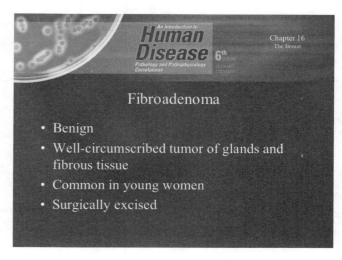

Fibroadenoma

- Benign
- Well-circumscribed tumor of glands and fibrous tissue
- Common in young women
- Surgically excised

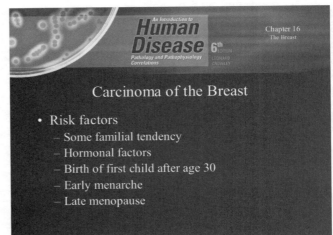

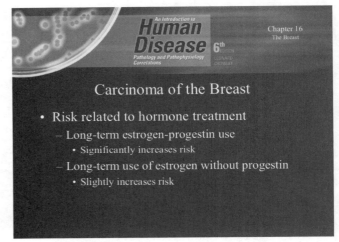

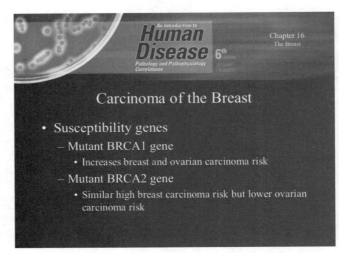

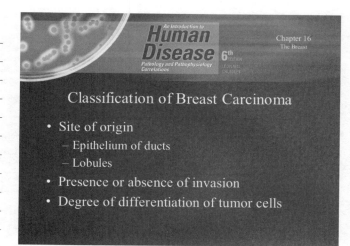

Classification of Breast Carcinoma

- Site of origin
  - Epithelium of ducts
  - Lobules
- Presence or absence of invasion
- Degree of differentiation of tumor cells

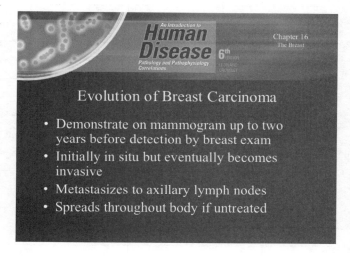

Evolution of Breast Carcinoma

- Demonstrate on mammogram up to two years before detection by breast exam
- Initially in situ but eventually becomes invasive
- Metastasizes to axillary lymph nodes
- Spreads throughout body if untreated

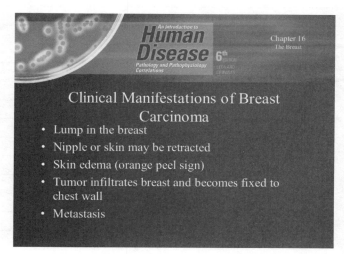

Clinical Manifestations of Breast Carcinoma

- Lump in the breast
- Nipple or skin may be retracted
- Skin edema (orange peel sign)
- Tumor infiltrates breast and becomes fixed to chest wall
- Metastasis

Notes

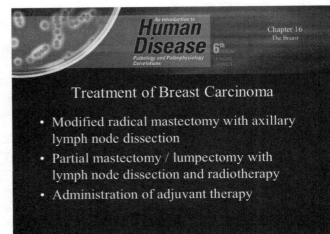

Treatment of Breast Carcinoma

- Modified radical mastectomy with axillary lymph node dissection
- Partial mastectomy / lumpectomy with lymph node dissection and radiotherapy
- Administration of adjuvant therapy

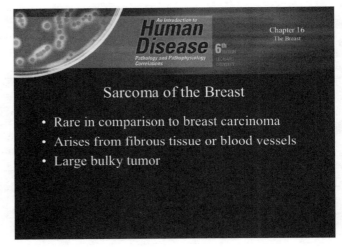

Sarcoma of the Breast

- Rare in comparison to breast carcinoma
- Arises from fibrous tissue or blood vessels
- Large bulky tumor

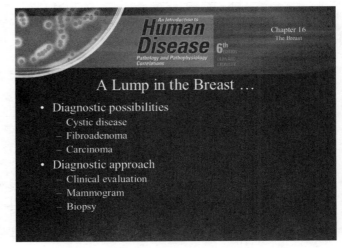

A Lump in the Breast …

- Diagnostic possibilities
  - Cystic disease
  - Fibroadenoma
  - Carcinoma
- Diagnostic approach
  - Clinical evaluation
  - Mammogram
  - Biopsy

Chapter Outline

The chapter outline provides you with an organizational guide to the topics and ideas presented in this chapter of the text.

Infections of the Female Genital Tract
    Vaginitis
    Cervicitis
    Salpingitis and Pelvic Inflammatory Disease
    Condylomas of the Genital Tract
Endometriosis
Cervical Polyps
Cervical Dysplasia and Cervical Carcinoma
    Diagnosis and Treatment
Endometrial Hyperplasia, Polyps, and Carcinoma
Uterine Myomas
Irregular Uterine Bleeding
    Dysfunctional Uterine Bleeding
    Other Causes of Uterine Bleeding
    Diagnosis and Treatment
Dysmenorrhea
Cysts and Tumors of the Ovary
Diseases of the Vulva
    Vulvar Dystrophy
    Carcinoma of the Vulva
Toxic Shock Syndrome
Contraception
Effects of Prenatal Exposure to Diethylstilbestrol (DES)

Study Questions

The following questions are provided as a test for comprehension and as a study guide for use with the text chapters. Additional study material is located at http://health.jbpub.com/humandisease/, which contains useful eLearning tools such as an A&P review, animated flashcards, interactive online glossary, crossword puzzles, and Web links.

Key Terms

Define the following terms:

1. Endometriosis _____

2. Toxic shock syndrome _____

3. Dysfunctional uterine bleeding _____

4. Dysmenorrhea _____

Fill-in-the-Blank

1. Warty overgrowths of genital tract squamous epithelium are caused by _____ and are called

    _____.

2. Abnormal, disorderly proliferation of cervical squamous epithelium is called _____.

3. A common benign uterine tumor is called a _____.

4. Cramp-like abdominal discomfort related to menstruation is called _____.

5. The cell that gives rise to a benign cystic ovarian teratoma (dermoid cyst) is _____.

6. An estrogen-producing tumor arising from the follicular cells (granulosa cells) lining an ovarian follicle is

    called a _____.

7. The organism responsible for toxic shock syndrome is _____.

8. The condition in which endometrium is found in locations outside the endometrial lining of the uterus is

    called _____.

True/False

1. Tell whether each statement is true or false regarding estrogen-progestin contraceptive pills. If false, explain why the statement is incorrect.

    a. These pills prevent ovulation. _____

    _____

    b. They may predispose a woman to tubal pregnancies. _____

    _____

    c. They may promote development of endometriosis. _____

    _____

    d. They may lead to thromboembolic complications in susceptible individuals. _____

    _____

e. The risk of pill-related complications is lower in cigarette smokers. _____

_____

2. Tell whether each statement is true or false regarding human papillomavirus (HPV). If false, explain why the statement is incorrect.

   a. Only a few types of HPV can infect the cervix. _____

   _____

   b. Most HPV types are carcinogenic (cancer causing). _____

   _____

   c. Most HPV infections cannot be eradicated by the body's immune defenses and become chronic. _____

   _____

   d. Testing cervical material obtained by a Pap smear for HPV may be a useful supplementary test when atypical cells are identified in the Pap smear. _____

   _____

Identify

1. Identify the organisms responsible for the three common causes of vaginitis.

   a. _____
   b. _____
   c. _____

2. A woman consults her physician because of irregular uterine bleeding. Identify five possible causes of uterine bleeding.

   a. _____
   b. _____
   c. _____
   d. _____
   e. _____

Discussion Questions

1. A woman has a human papillomavirus (HPV) infection of her cervical epithelium. What factors influence her risk of developing cervical dysplasia or in situ carcinoma? _____

   _____

   _____

   _____

2. If a woman is 65 years old and has irregular uterine bleeding, what is the likely cause of the bleeding? _____
_____
_____
_____

3. What are the clinical features of toxic shock syndrome in a menstruating woman? _____
_____
_____
_____

4. Describe how contraceptive pills function to prevent pregnancy. _____
_____
_____
_____

5. What are the manifestations and complications of endometriosis? _____
_____
_____
_____

6. What parts of the female genital tract may be involved in gonorrheal infection? _____
_____
_____
_____

7. How does gonorrhea lead to sterility? _____
_____
_____
_____

8. What is the difference between in situ and invasive cervical carcinoma? How is the Pap smear used in the diagnosis of carcinoma? _____
_____
_____
_____

9. Explain whether the following conditions may predispose susceptible individuals to toxic shock syndrome.
   a. Use of tampons _____
   _____
   b. Use of a vaginal (contraceptive) diaphragm _____
   _____

c. Use of contraceptive sponges _____

_____

d. Use of an IUD _____

_____

e. Use of contraceptive foam and condoms _____

_____

10. A patient has dysmenorrhea and endometriosis is suspected. What diagnostic procedures are helpful in establishing a diagnosis of this condition? _____

_____

_____

_____

11. A 62-year-old woman has irregular vaginal bleeding. What conditions could account for this condition? _____

_____

_____

_____

CERVICITIS

NON SPECIFIC
SPECIFIC
- CHLAMYDIA
- GONORRHEA

CERVICAL NEOPLASIA

DYSPLASIA-IN SITU CA (CIN)
INVASIVE CARCINOMA

UTERINE DISEASES

ENDOMETRIAL
    HYPERPLASIA
    POLYP
    CARCINOMA

TOXIC
SHOCK
SYNDROME

OVARY DISEASES

FUNCTIONAL CYSTS
CYSTIC TUMORS
    - BENIGN
    - MALIGNANT
SOLID TUMORS
    - BENIGN
    - MALIGNANT

ENDOMETRIOSIS

ECTOPIC ENDOMETRIUM
IN PELVIS.

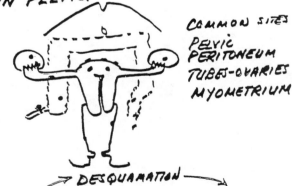

COMMON SITES
PELVIC
PERITONEUM
TUBES-OVARIES
MYOMETRIUM

CYCLIC CHANGE → DESQUAMATION → (PAIN) → INFLAMMATION → SCARRING

ETIOLOGY
COMPLICATIONS
TREATMENT

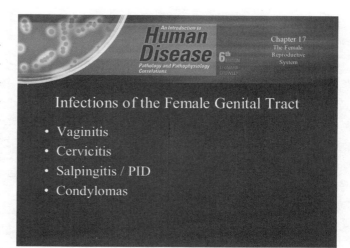

Infections of the Female Genital Tract

- Vaginitis
- Cervicitis
- Salpingitis / PID
- Condylomas

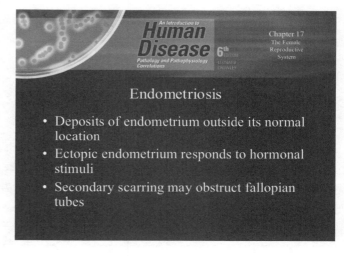

Endometriosis

- Deposits of endometrium outside its normal location
- Ectopic endometrium responds to hormonal stimuli
- Secondary scarring may obstruct fallopian tubes

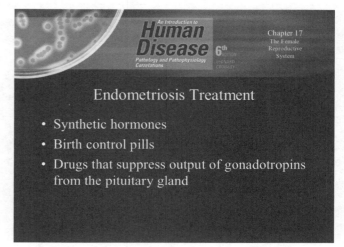

Endometriosis Treatment

- Synthetic hormones
- Birth control pills
- Drugs that suppress output of gonadotropins from the pituitary gland

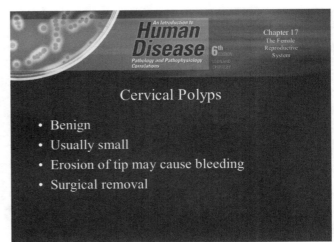

Cervical Polyps

- Benign
- Usually small
- Erosion of tip may cause bleeding
- Surgical removal

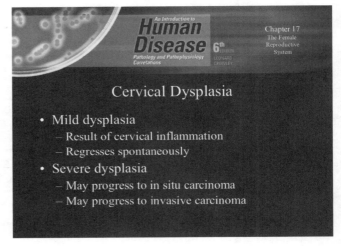

Cervical Dysplasia

- Mild dysplasia
  - Result of cervical inflammation
  - Regresses spontaneously
- Severe dysplasia
  - May progress to in situ carcinoma
  - May progress to invasive carcinoma

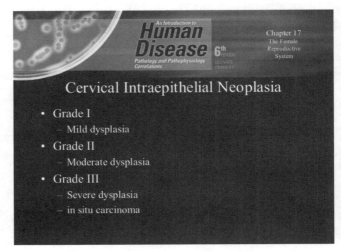

Cervical Intraepithelial Neoplasia

- Grade I
  - Mild dysplasia
- Grade II
  - Moderate dysplasia
- Grade III
  - Severe dysplasia
  - in situ carcinoma

Notes

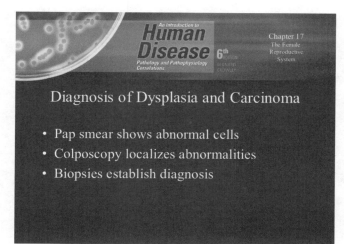

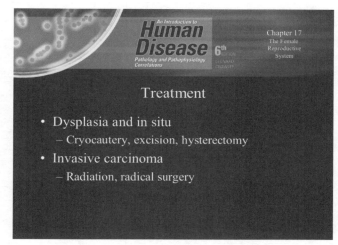

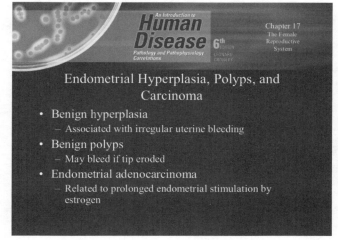

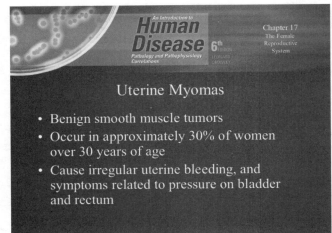

Uterine Myomas

- Benign smooth muscle tumors
- Occur in approximately 30% of women over 30 years of age
- Cause irregular uterine bleeding, and symptoms related to pressure on bladder and rectum

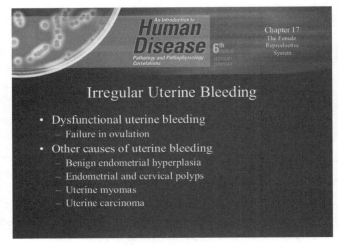

Irregular Uterine Bleeding

- Dysfunctional uterine bleeding
  - Failure in ovulation
- Other causes of uterine bleeding
  - Benign endometrial hyperplasia
  - Endometrial and cervical polyps
  - Uterine myomas
  - Uterine carcinoma

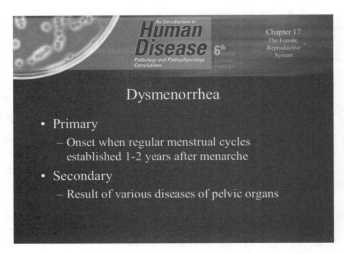

Dysmenorrhea

- Primary
  - Onset when regular menstrual cycles established 1-2 years after menarche
- Secondary
  - Result of various diseases of pelvic organs

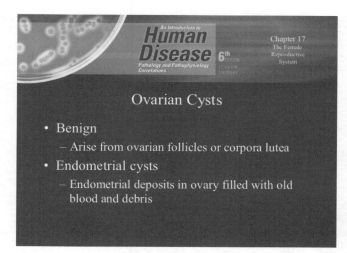

Ovarian Cysts

- Benign
  - Arise from ovarian follicles or corpora lutea
- Endometrial cysts
  - Endometrial deposits in ovary filled with old blood and debris

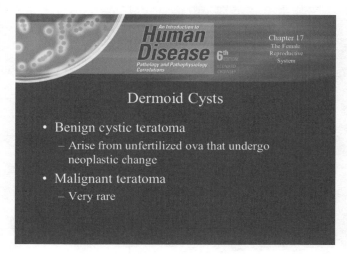

Dermoid Cysts

- Benign cystic teratoma
  - Arise from unfertilized ova that undergo neoplastic change
- Malignant teratoma
  - Very rare

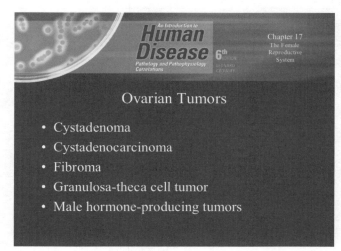

Ovarian Tumors

- Cystadenoma
- Cystadenocarcinoma
- Fibroma
- Granulosa-theca cell tumor
- Male hormone-producing tumors

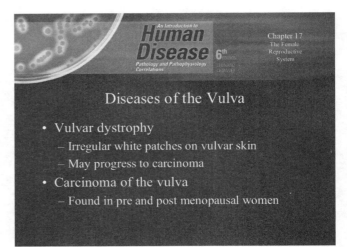

Diseases of the Vulva

- Vulvar dystrophy
  - Irregular white patches on vulvar skin
  - May progress to carcinoma
- Carcinoma of the vulva
  - Found in pre and post menopausal women

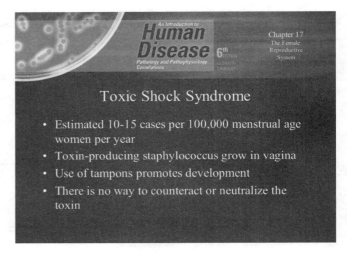

Toxic Shock Syndrome

- Estimated 10-15 cases per 100,000 menstrual age women per year
- Toxin-producing staphylococcus grow in vagina
- Use of tampons promotes development
- There is no way to counteract or neutralize the toxin

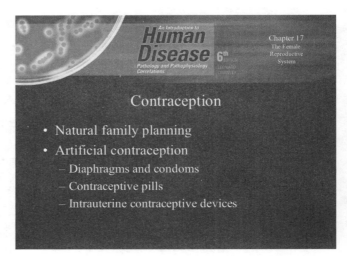

Contraception

- Natural family planning
- Artificial contraception
  - Diaphragms and condoms
  - Contraceptive pills
  - Intrauterine contraceptive devices

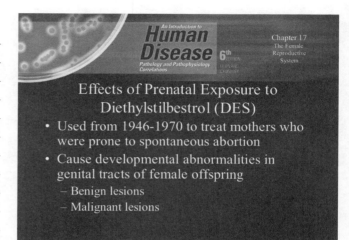

Chapter 18 Prenatal Development and Diseases Associated with Pregnancy

Chapter Outline

The chapter outline provides you with an organizational guide to the topics and ideas presented in this chapter of the text.

Study Questions

The following questions are provided as a test for comprehension and as a study guide for use with the text chapters. Additional study material is located at http://health.jbpub.com/humandisease/, which contains useful eLearning tools such as an A&P review, animated flashcards, interactive online glossary, crossword puzzles, and Web links.

Key Terms

Define the following terms:

1. Amniotic fluid _____

2. Gestational trophoblast disease _____

3. Placenta _____

4. Rh immune globulin _____

Fill-in-the-Blank

1. In a woman with a regular 28-day menstrual cycle, ovulation normally occurs on day _____.

2. If the egg is fertilized, its implantation occurs _____ days after fertilization occurs.

3. During the _____ period, the developing organism is most vulnerable to injury from drugs, maternal infections, or other factors that disturb prenatal development.

4. The outer sac surrounding the embryo is called the _____, and the finger-like processes projecting from the sac are called _____.

5. In the placenta, the blood circulating through the villi is blood pumped into the placenta by the _____, and the blood flowing around the villi is blood pumped into the placenta by _____.

6. An excess of amnionic fluid is called _____.

7. A reduced volume of amnionic fluid is called _____. This condition may be caused by _____.

8. The condition in which the placenta attaches to the lower part of the uterus and covers the cervix is called _____. This condition is usually treated by _____.

9. Identical twins are formed by separation of the inner cell mass during the early stages of prenatal development. If the separation is incomplete, the result is _____.

10. If the placental circulations of identical twins are interconnected, one twin may become anemic and the other twin will have an excessive amount of blood. This condition is called _____.

11. The placenta produces two steroid hormones, called _____ and _____. It also produces two protein hormones, called _____ and _____.

12. In the usual case of hemolytic disease caused by Rh incompatibility, the Rh (D) type of the father is _____. The infant's Rh type is _____, and the mother's Rh type is _____.

True/False

Tell whether each statement is true or false. If false, explain why the statement is incorrect.

1. Two Rh-negative parents may have an Rh-positive infant. _____

   _____

2. An Rh-negative infant may be born to two Rh-positive parents. _____

   _____

3. Rh immune globulin is sometimes administered to Rh-negative mothers during pregnancy. _____

   _____

4. Rh hemolytic disease usually occurs in firstborn infants and is usually less severe in subsequent pregnancies.

   _____

5. Tell whether each statement is true or false regarding hydatidiform mole. If false, explain why the statement is incorrect.

   a. It occurs less frequently in U.S. and Canadian women than in women living in Asia. _____

      _____

   b. Incomplete removal of a hydatidiform mole may be followed by development of a choriocarcinoma. _____

      _____

   c. A woman who has had a mole evacuated by curettage may attempt another pregnancy as soon as her normal

      menstrual periods resume after the curettage. _____

      _____

   d. Some moles may exhibit aggressive behavior and invade the uterine wall. _____

      _____

6. Tell whether each statement is true or false regarding Rh immune globulin. If false, explain why the statement is incorrect.

   a. Its administration will usually prevent sensitization of an Rh-negative mother who has given birth to an

      Rh-positive infant. _____

      _____

   b. Its administration will usually prevent ABO hemolytic disease in group O mothers who have given birth to

      group A or B infants. _____

      _____

   c. Its administration will reduce the concentration of preexisting Rh antibodies in an Rh-negative mother who has

      previously been sensitized to the Rh antigen. _____

      _____

   d. It is never given to Rh-positive infants born to Rh-negative mothers. _____

      _____

Identify

1. Prenatal development is divided into three separate periods:

   a. _____

   b. _____

   c. _____

2. List the two conditions that may lead to the excess amniotic fluid.

   a. _____

   b. _____

3. The term "gestational trophoblast disease" includes what three conditions?

   a. _____

   b. _____

   c. _____

Discussion Questions

1. In what part of the genital tract does fertilization of the egg occur? _____

   _____

   _____

   _____

2. Briefly describe how gestational trophoblast disease is treated, and how the patient should be managed after the condition is treated. _____

   _____

   _____

   _____

3. Normally maternal and fetal blood do not intermix in the placenta when the intact placenta remains within the uterus. How does this situation change when the placenta separates from the uterus after the baby has been delivered?

   _____

   _____

   _____

4. Postpartum administration of Rh immune globulin to an Rh-negative woman who has given birth to an Rh-positive infant is recommended and given routinely to such patients. What is the purpose of the injection, and why is it effective? _____

   _____

   _____

   _____

5. Can two Rh (D)-negative parents have an Rh-positive baby? Why or why not? _____

_____

_____

_____

6. Can two Rh (D)-positive parents have an Rh-negative baby? Why or why not? _____

_____

_____

_____

7. Describe how ABO hemolytic disease differs from Rh hemolytic disease. _____

_____

_____

_____

8. Why do spontaneous abortions occur? _____

_____

_____

_____

9. What are the consequences of prolonged retention of a dead fetus within the uterine cavity? _____

_____

_____

_____

10. What is an ectopic pregnancy? What factors predispose a woman to development of an ectopic pregnancy in the

fallopian tube? What are the consequences of a tubal pregnancy? _____

_____

_____

_____

11. What conditions are associated with ectopic pregnancies? _____

_____

_____

_____

12. Who should receive the Rh immune globulin injection? When is it given? Why is it given? How does it work?

_____

_____

_____

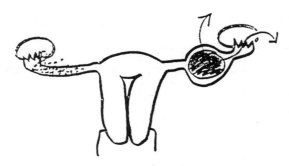

INFLAMMATION

TUBE AND ADNEXA (PID)
- CHLAMYDIA
- GONOCOCCUS
- OTHER ORGANISMS

ECTOPIC PREGNANCY
- SITES
- PREDISPOSING FACTORS
- SIGNIFICANCE

GESTATIONAL TROPHOBLAST DISEASE RESULTS FROM ABNORMAL CONCEPTION

HYDATIDIFORM MOLE
COMPLETE
PARTIAL
INVASIVE MOLE
CHORIOCARCINOMA

MANIFESTATIONS
- SIZE OF UTERUS DOESN'T MATCH STAGE OF PREGNANCY
- BLEEDING AND EXPULSION OF MOLAR TISSUE
- ABNORMAL ULTRASOUND
- CHORIOCARCINOMA IS MOST AGGRESSIVE TYPE AND MAY FOLLOW INCOMPLETE REMOVAL OF MOLE

TREATMENT
- EVACUATE MOLE AND FOLLOW HCG LEVEL (HYSTERECTOMY OK IN OLDER WOMAN)
- CHEMOTHERAPY IF MOLE RECURS
- NO PREGANCY FOR ONE YEAR

FERTILIZE   DIVIDE   IMPLANT

TWINS

IDENTICAL	FRATERNAL
30%	70%

PLACENTAL STRUCTURE
DiDi   70% FRATERNAL
        30% IDENTICAL

DIAMNIONIC
MONOCHORIONIC } ALWAYS IDENTICAL
MONO/MONO

PROBLEMS
1. OVERLOADED UTERUS
2. TWIN TRANSFUSION SYNDROME
3. CONJOINED

"VANISHING TWINS"

MANAGEMENT

MONITOR PATIENT AT RISK

PREVENT SENSITIZATION
- RH IMMUNE GLOBULIN

POSTPARTUM - 1.5% SENSITIZATION

ANTEPARTUM
AND POSTPARTUM - 0.15%

(NO RHOGAM 15%)

MONITOR SENSITIZED PATIENT

AMNIOCENTESIS
PRETERM DELIVERY
CONTROL ANEMIA / HIGH BILIRUBIN
AFTER DELIVERY

INTRAUTERINE TRANSFUSION
IN SEVERELY AFFECTED INFANT

HEMOLYTIC DISEASE

1. BLOOD GROUP INCOMPATIBLE
MATING (INFANT HAS ANTIGEN
MOTHER LACKS)

2. INFANT SENSITIZES MOTHER
(INFANTS CELLS GET INTO MOTHERS
CIRCULATION)

3. MOTHER FORMS ANTIBODY

4. ANTIBODY CROSSES PLACENTA
DAMAGES INFANTS CELLS
(HEMOLYSIS)

5. INFANT ATTEMPTS TO "KEEP UP"
WITH INCREASED BLOOD DESTRUCTION

OUTCOME

1. MILD / MODERATE - LIVEBORN
ANEMIA / JAUNDICE
(GETS WORSE AFTER DELIVERY)

2. SEVERE - INTRAUTERINE DEATH
ANEMIA / HYDROPS / JAUNDICE

ABO HEMOLYTIC DISEASE

```
┌──────────┐        ┌──────────────┐
│ A OR B   │        │ GROUP O      │
│ INFANT   │        │ MOTHER       │
│          │        │ (HAS ANTI-A  │
│          │        │  ANTI-B      │
└──────────┘        └──────────────┘
```

ANTIGENIC STIMULATION

RISE AND CHANGE IN MATERNAL ANTIBODY

MILD DISEASE
FIRST PREGNANCY
MAY NOT REQUIRE TREATMENT

ABO INCOMPATIBILITY PROTECTS
RH NEGATIVE MOTHER FROM RH
HEMOLYTIC DISEASE.   WHY?

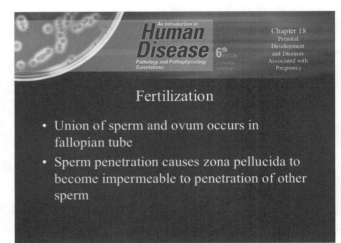

Fertilization

- Union of sperm and ovum occurs in fallopian tube
- Sperm penetration causes zona pellucida to become impermeable to penetration of other sperm

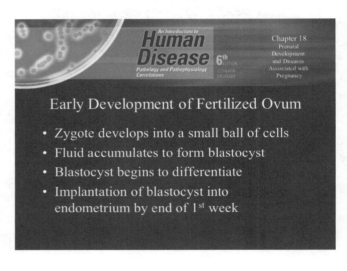

Early Development of Fertilized Ovum

- Zygote develops into a small ball of cells
- Fluid accumulates to form blastocyst
- Blastocyst begins to differentiate
- Implantation of blastocyst into endometrium by end of 1st week

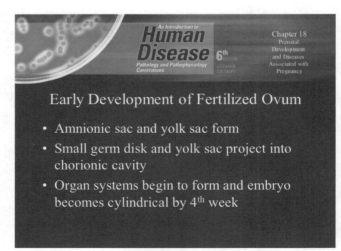

Early Development of Fertilized Ovum

- Amnionic sac and yolk sac form
- Small germ disk and yolk sac project into chorionic cavity
- Organ systems begin to form and embryo becomes cylindrical by 4th week

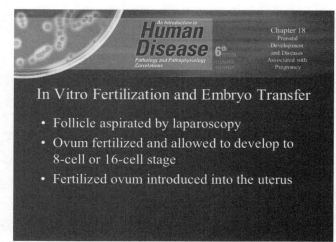

In Vitro Fertilization and Embryo Transfer

- Follicle aspirated by laparoscopy
- Ovum fertilized and allowed to develop to 8-cell or 16-cell stage
- Fertilized ovum introduced into the uterus

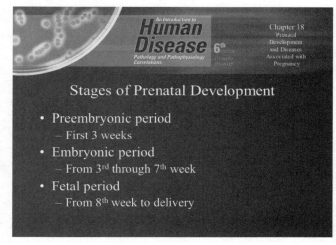

Stages of Prenatal Development

- Preembryonic period
  - First 3 weeks
- Embryonic period
  - From 3rd through 7th week
- Fetal period
  - From 8th week to delivery

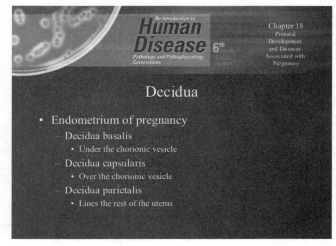

Decidua

- Endometrium of pregnancy
  - Decidua basalis
    - Under the chorionic vesicle
  - Decidua capsularis
    - Over the chorionic vesicle
  - Decidua parietalis
    - Lines the rest of the uterus

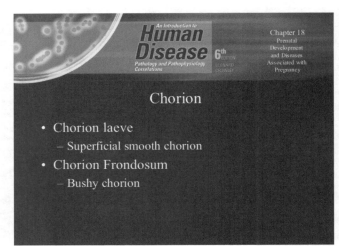

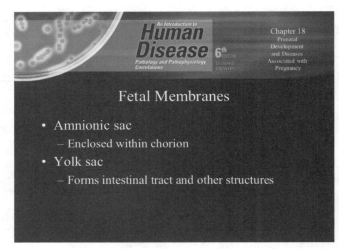

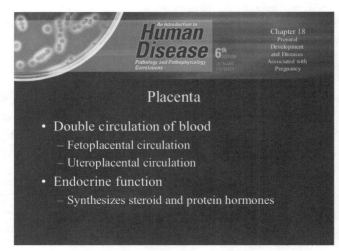

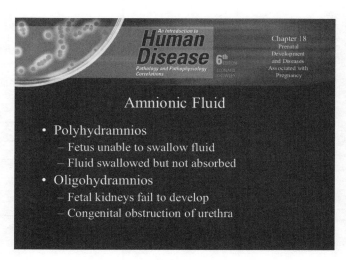

Amnionic Fluid

- Polyhydramnios
  - Fetus unable to swallow fluid
  - Fluid swallowed but not absorbed
- Oligohydramnios
  - Fetal kidneys fail to develop
  - Congenital obstruction of urethra

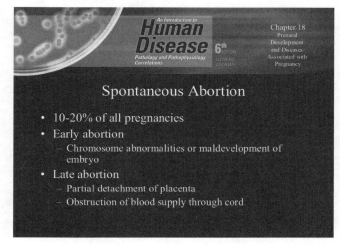

Spontaneous Abortion

- 10-20% of all pregnancies
- Early abortion
  - Chromosome abnormalities or maldevelopment of embryo
- Late abortion
  - Partial detachment of placenta
  - Obstruction of blood supply through cord

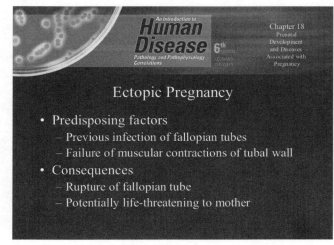

Ectopic Pregnancy

- Predisposing factors
  - Previous infection of fallopian tubes
  - Failure of muscular contractions of tubal wall
- Consequences
  - Rupture of fallopian tube
  - Potentially life-threatening to mother

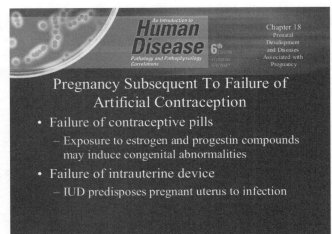

Pregnancy Subsequent To Failure of Artificial Contraception

- Failure of contraceptive pills
  - Exposure to estrogen and progestin compounds may induce congenital abnormalities
- Failure of intrauterine device
  - IUD predisposes pregnant uterus to infection

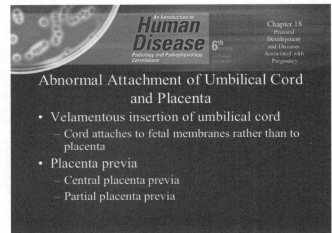

Abnormal Attachment of Umbilical Cord and Placenta

- Velamentous insertion of umbilical cord
  - Cord attaches to fetal membranes rather than to placenta
- Placenta previa
  - Central placenta previa
  - Partial placenta previa

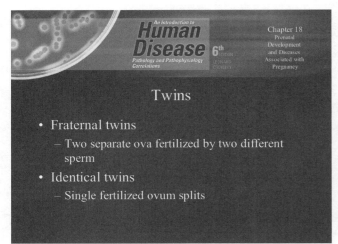

Twins

- Fraternal twins
  - Two separate ova fertilized by two different sperm
- Identical twins
  - Single fertilized ovum splits

Notes

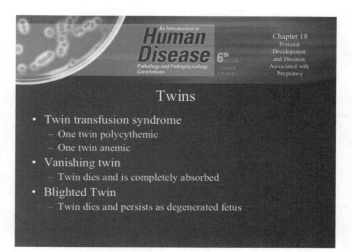

Twins

- Twin transfusion syndrome
  - One twin polycythemic
  - One twin anemic
- Vanishing twin
  - Twin dies and is completely absorbed
- Blighted Twin
  - Twin dies and persists as degenerated fetus

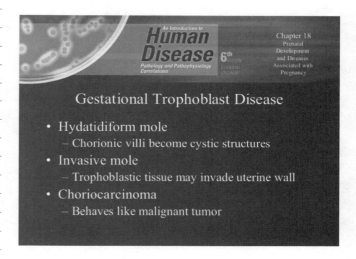

Gestational Trophoblast Disease

- Hydatidiform mole
  - Chorionic villi become cystic structures
- Invasive mole
  - Trophoblastic tissue may invade uterine wall
- Choriocarcinoma
  - Behaves like malignant tumor

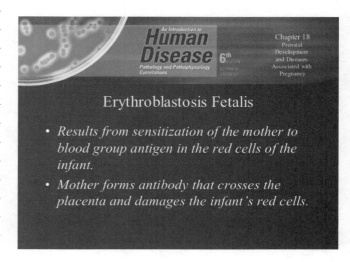

Erythroblastosis Fetalis

- *Results from sensitization of the mother to blood group antigen in the red cells of the infant.*
- *Mother forms antibody that crosses the placenta and damages the infant's red cells.*

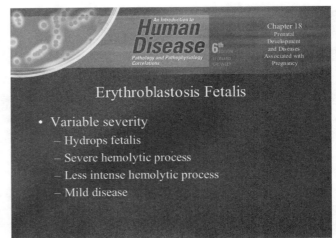

Erythroblastosis Fetalis

- Variable severity
  - Hydrops fetalis
  - Severe hemolytic process
  - Less intense hemolytic process
  - Mild disease

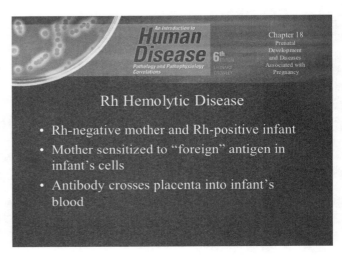

Rh Hemolytic Disease

- Rh-negative mother and Rh-positive infant
- Mother sensitized to "foreign" antigen in infant's cells
- Antibody crosses placenta into infant's blood

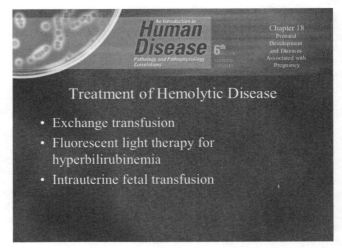

Treatment of Hemolytic Disease

- Exchange transfusion
- Fluorescent light therapy for hyperbilirubinemia
- Intrauterine fetal transfusion

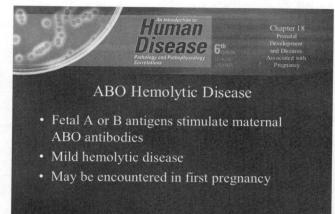

ABO Hemolytic Disease

- Fetal A or B antigens stimulate maternal ABO antibodies
- Mild hemolytic disease
- May be encountered in first pregnancy

Chapter Outline

The chapter outline provides you with an organizational guide to the topics and ideas presented in this chapter of the text.

Study Questions

The following questions are provided as a test for comprehension and as a study guide for use with the text chapters. Additional study material is located at http://health.jbpub.com/humandisease/, which contains useful eLearning tools such as an A&P review, animated flashcards, interactive online glossary, crossword puzzles, and Web links.

Key Terms

Define the following terms:

1. Diabetic nephropathy _____

2. Urea _____

3. Uremia _____

4. Glomerulonephritis _____

5. Pyelonephritis _____

6. Nephritic syndrome _____

7. Nephrosclerosis _____

Fill-in-the-Blank

1. The enzyme released by juxtaglomerular cells is called _____ , which converts a protein called _____ into _____. The converted protein then is converted by ACE into _____, which is a powerful vasoconstrictor and also stimulates the adrenal cortex to release a hormone called _____.

2. Glomerulonephritis results from an immunologic reaction within the glomeruli, and is divided into two main types, which are called _____ and _____.

3. An infection of the bladder is called _____, and an infection of the kidney is called _____.

4. Dilatation of the renal pelvis, calyces, and ureter resulting from obstruction to outflow of urine is called _____.

5. A kidney stone is called a _____.

6. The hereditary kidney disease characterized by formation of multiple progressively enlarging renal cysts that gradually destroy the function of the kidneys is called _____.

7. Two methods of renal dialysis are called _____ and _____.

8. Malignant tumors occur in the kidneys and bladder. The malignant kidney tumor occurring in older adults is called _____. The malignant kidney tumor occurring in infants and young children is called _____. The malignant bladder tumor is called _____.

9. The laboratory test that is likely to show abnormal results in a patient with acute glomerulonephritis is _____.

True/False

Tell whether each statement is true or false. If false, explain why the statement is incorrect.

1. Blood and urine clearance tests measure the ability of the kidneys to remove ("clear") waste products from the blood and excrete the products in the urine. _____

_____

2. Diabetic nephropathy is characterized by nodular and diffuse thickening of glomerular basement membranes as well as by marked thickening and narrowing of glomerular arterioles (arteriolonephrosclerosis). _____

_____

3. Tell whether each statement is true or false regarding acute post-streptococcal glomerulonephritis. If false, explain why the statement is incorrect.

   a. It is induced by antigen–antibody complexes filtered from the blood that accumulate within the walls of the glomerular capillaries. _____

   _____

   b. It results from bacterial infection of the glomeruli. _____

   _____

   c. It usually causes a nephrotic syndrome. _____

   _____

   d. It is caused by damage done by enzymes released from leukocytes that accumulate within the glomeruli.

   _____

4. Tell whether each statement is true or false regarding the nephrotic syndrome. If false, explain why the statement is incorrect.

   a. The liver fails to produce plasma protein. _____

   _____

   b. Protein is lost in the urine more rapidly than it can be produced by the body. _____

   _____

   c. The nephrotic syndrome is usually associated with normal concentration of plasma protein and normal plasma osmotic pressure. _____

   _____

   d. It may result from any type of glomerular disease that allows large amounts of protein to escape in the urine.

   _____

   e. It usually results in bacterial infection of the kidney. _____

   _____

   f. It may result from renal tubular disease. _____

   _____

5. Tell whether each statement is true or false regarding the renin-angiotensin-aldosterone syndrome. If false, explain why the statement is incorrect.

   a. Renin is secreted by cells of the juxtaglomerular apparatus in response to high blood sodium concentration, higher-than-normal blood pressure, or higher-than-normal blood volume. _____

   _____

   b. Renin converts angiotensinogen to angiotensin I. _____

   _____

   c. Angiotensin-converting enzyme (ACE) converts angiotensin I to angiotensin II. _____

   _____

   d. Angiotensin II stimulates aldosterone release and arteriolar vasoconstriction. _____

   _____

6. Tell whether each statement is true or false regarding congenital polycystic kidney disease. If false, explain why the statement is incorrect.

   a. It is transmitted as mendelian dominant trait. _____

   _____

   b. Manifestations occur in late childhood or adolescence. _____

   _____

   c. Progressively enlarging cysts slowly destroy kidney function. _____

   _____

   d. Affected kidneys become greatly enlarged. _____

   _____

7. Tell whether each statement is true or false regarding bladder carcinoma. If false, explain why the statement is incorrect.

   a. The bladder tumor arises from transitional epithelium of the urinary bladder. _____

   _____

   b. Hematuria (blood in urine) may be the first manifestation of the bladder tumor. _____

   _____

   c. The tumor usually is poorly differentiated and rapidly growing, and has a very poor prognosis. _____

   _____

   d. Diagnosis of a tumor is made by cystoscopy and biopsy. _____

   _____

Identify

1. Identify three conditions that predispose a person to urinary tract infection.

   a. _____

   b. _____

   c. _____

2. Identify three features characteristic of the nephrotic syndrome.

   a. _____

   b. _____

   c. _____

Discussion Questions

1. What is the relationship between glomerulonephritis and beta streptococcal infection? _____

   _____

   _____

   _____

2. What is the difference between the nephrotic syndrome and nephrosclerosis? _____

   _____

   _____

   _____

3. Why does edema occur in a patient with nephrosis? _____

   _____

   _____

   _____

4. What are the common causes of urinary tract obstruction? What are its effects on the kidneys and lower urinary tract?

   _____

   _____

   _____

5. What conditions predispose a person to kidney stones? _____

   _____

   _____

   _____

6. Describe the conditions that may lead to renal tubular necrosis. What are its clinical manifestations? _____

   _____

   _____

   _____

7. What is the significance of an elevated level of urea in the blood? _____

_____

_____

_____

8. What are the manifestations of uremia? How is it treated by the physician? _____

_____

_____

_____

9. How is kidney failure treated? _____

_____

_____

_____

10. What methods does the physician use to establish a diagnosis of renal disease? _____

_____

_____

_____

11. What condition(s) may eventually lead to renal failure? _____

_____

_____

_____

12. What adverse effects are caused by a foreign body inserted into the bladder? _____

_____

_____

_____

13. What factors predispose a person to the formation of calculi in the urinary tract? _____

_____

_____

_____

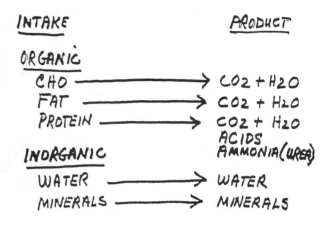

INTAKE	PRODUCT
ORGANIC	
CHO	$\longrightarrow$ $CO_2 + H_2O$
FAT	$\longrightarrow$ $CO_2 + H_2O$
PROTEIN	$\longrightarrow$ $CO_2 + H_2O$
	ACIDS
	AMMONIA (UREA)
INORGANIC	
WATER	$\longrightarrow$ WATER
MINERALS	$\longrightarrow$ MINERALS

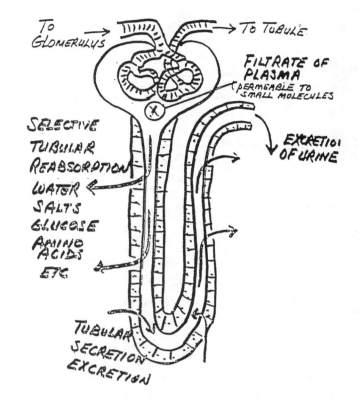

NORMAL FUNCTION REQUIRES

1. FREE FLOW OF BLOOD THROUGH AFFERENT GLOMERULAR ARTERIOLE

2. NORMAL GLOMERULAR CAPILLARIES

3. NORMAL FILTERING MEMBRANE

4. INTACT TUBULE

5. NORMAL URINARY DRAINAGE

GLOMERULONEPHRITIS	— IMMUNOLOGIC INJURY
NEPHROSIS	LEAKY FILTER WITH LARGE PROTEIN LOSS
PYELONEPHRITIS	BACTERIAL INFECTION
HYDRONEPHROSIS	URINARY TRACT OBSTRUCTION
TUBULAR NECROSIS	CHEMICAL OR VASCULAR INJURY
STONES (CALCULI)	DISTURBED SOLUBILITY OF CONSTITUENTS
FOREIGN BODIES	MUCOSAL INJURY
NEPHROSCEROSIS — DIFFUSE — NODULAR	GLOMERULAR VASCULAR LESIONS.

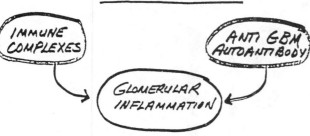

IMMUNE COMPLEXES

ANTI GBM AUTOANTIBODY

GLOMERULAR INFLAMMATION

MILD ⟶ SEVERE

RECOVERY   LOSS OF RENAL FUNCTION

NEPHROSIS
(NEPHROTIC SYNDROME)

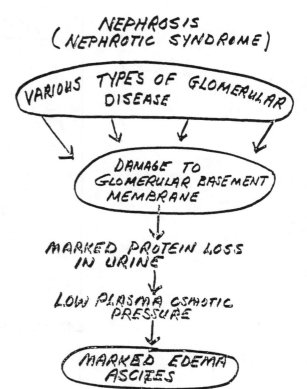

VARIOUS TYPES OF GLOMERULAR DISEASE

DAMAGE TO GLOMERULAR BASEMENT MEMBRANE

MARKED PROTEIN LOSS IN URINE

LOW PLASMA OSMOTIC PRESSURE

MARKED EDEMA ASCITES

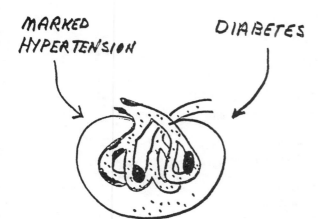

MARKED HYPERTENSION   DIABETES

ARTERIOLONEPHROSCLEROSIS

DIABETIC GLOMERULOSCLEROSIS

CYSTITIS

PYELONEPHRITIS

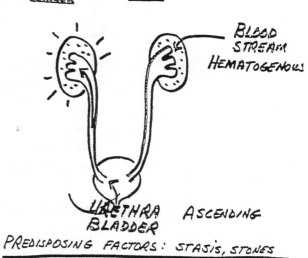

BLOOD STREAM HEMATOGENOUS

URETHRA   ASCENDING
BLADDER

PREDISPOSING FACTORS: STASIS, STONES

INFECTION

STASIS   STONES

HYDRONEPHROSIS

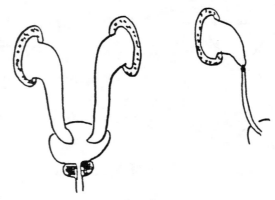

CAUSE: OBSTRUCTION
EFFECT: DISTENTION PROXIMAL
COMPLICATIONS: INFECTION
                    STONES
                    RENAL PRESSURE
                       ATROPHY

RENAL FAILURE

INSUFFICIENT FUNCTIONING RENAL TISSUE

RETENTION OF   CLINICAL
"WASTE" PRODUCTS   MANIFESTATIONS

UREA   ACIDOSIS
CREATININE   ELECTROLYTE
ORGANIC ACIDS   DISTURBANCES
MINERALS   ANEMIA
                      CONVULSIONS
                      COMA

TREATMENT
DIET
DIALYSIS
TRANSPLANTATION

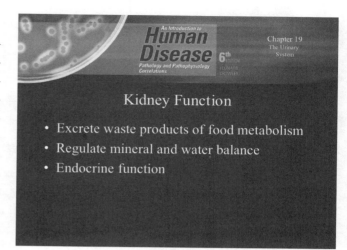

Kidney Function

- Excrete waste products of food metabolism
- Regulate mineral and water balance
- Endocrine function

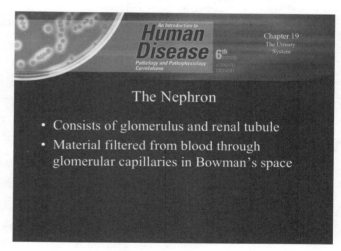

The Nephron

- Consists of glomerulus and renal tubule
- Material filtered from blood through glomerular capillaries in Bowman's space

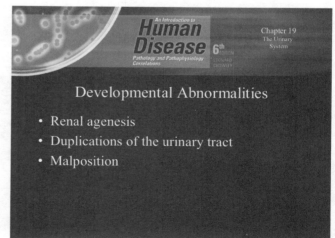

Developmental Abnormalities

- Renal agenesis
- Duplications of the urinary tract
- Malposition

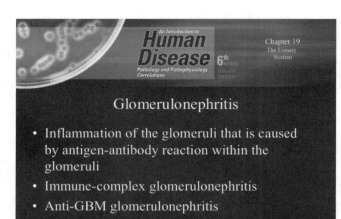

Glomerulonephritis

- Inflammation of the glomeruli that is caused by antigen-antibody reaction within the glomeruli
- Immune-complex glomerulonephritis
- Anti-GBM glomerulonephritis

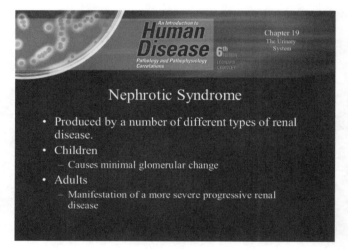

Nephrotic Syndrome

- Produced by a number of different types of renal disease.
- Children
  - Causes minimal glomerular change
- Adults
  - Manifestation of a more severe progressive renal disease

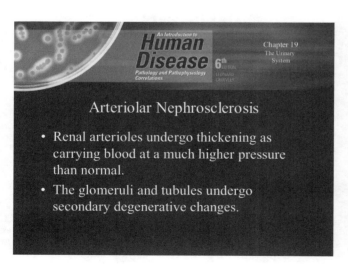

Arteriolar Nephrosclerosis

- Renal arterioles undergo thickening as carrying blood at a much higher pressure than normal.
- The glomeruli and tubules undergo secondary degenerative changes.

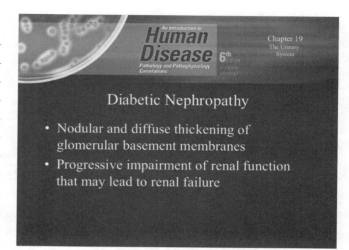

Diabetic Nephropathy

- Nodular and diffuse thickening of glomerular basement membranes
- Progressive impairment of renal function that may lead to renal failure

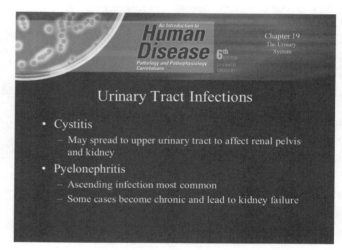

Urinary Tract Infections

- Cystitis
  - May spread to upper urinary tract to affect renal pelvis and kidney
- Pyelonephritis
  - Ascending infection most common
  - Some cases become chronic and lead to kidney failure

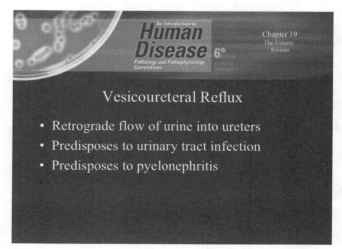

Vesicoureteral Reflux

- Retrograde flow of urine into ureters
- Predisposes to urinary tract infection
- Predisposes to pyelonephritis

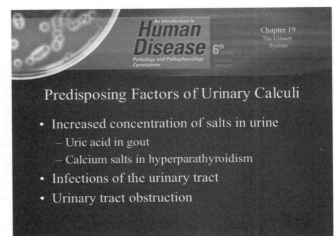

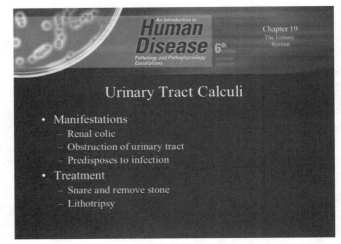

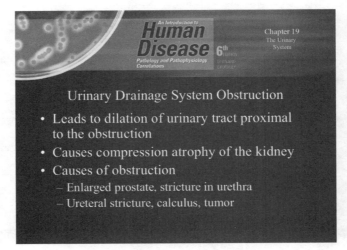

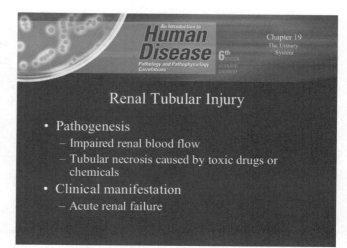

Renal Tubular Injury

- Pathogenesis
  - Impaired renal blood flow
  - Tubular necrosis caused by toxic drugs or chemicals
- Clinical manifestation
  - Acute renal failure

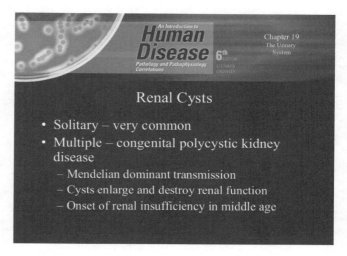

Renal Cysts

- Solitary – very common
- Multiple – congenital polycystic kidney disease
  - Mendelian dominant transmission
  - Cysts enlarge and destroy renal function
  - Onset of renal insufficiency in middle age

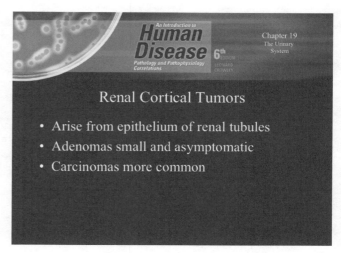

Renal Cortical Tumors

- Arise from epithelium of renal tubules
- Adenomas small and asymptomatic
- Carcinomas more common

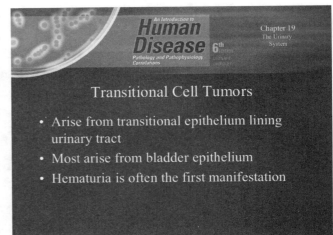

Transitional Cell Tumors

- Arise from transitional epithelium lining urinary tract
- Most arise from bladder epithelium
- Hematuria is often the first manifestation

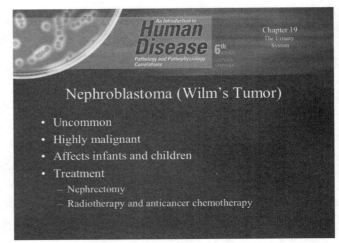

Nephroblastoma (Wilm's Tumor)

- Uncommon
- Highly malignant
- Affects infants and children
- Treatment
  - Nephrectomy
  - Radiotherapy and anticancer chemotherapy

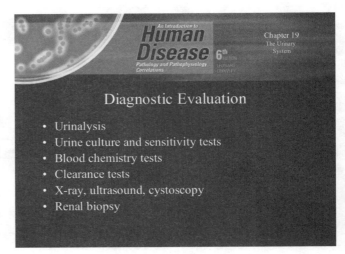

Diagnostic Evaluation

- Urinalysis
- Urine culture and sensitivity tests
- Blood chemistry tests
- Clearance tests
- X-ray, ultrasound, cystoscopy
- Renal biopsy

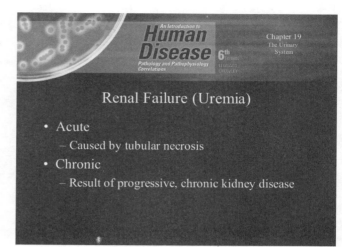

Renal Failure (Uremia)

- Acute
  - Caused by tubular necrosis
- Chronic
  - Result of progressive, chronic kidney disease

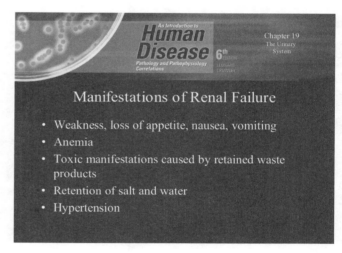

Manifestations of Renal Failure

- Weakness, loss of appetite, nausea, vomiting
- Anemia
- Toxic manifestations caused by retained waste products
- Retention of salt and water
- Hypertension

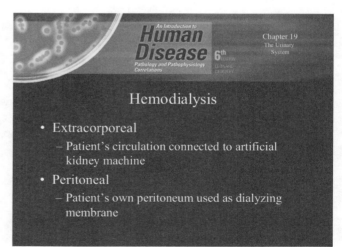

Hemodialysis

- Extracorporeal
  - Patient's circulation connected to artificial kidney machine
- Peritoneal
  - Patient's own peritoneum used as dialyzing membrane

_____

_____

_____

_____

_____

_____

_____

_____

_____

_____

_____

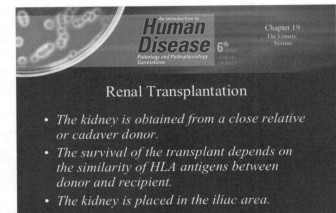

Renal Transplantation

- *The kidney is obtained from a close relative or cadaver donor.*
- *The survival of the transplant depends on the similarity of HLA antigens between donor and recipient.*
- *The kidney is placed in the iliac area.*

Chapter 20   The Male Reproductive System

Chapter Outline

The chapter outline provides you with an organizational guide to the topics and ideas presented in this chapter of the text.

Structure and Function of the Male Reproductive Organs
Gonorrhea and Nongonococcal Urethritis
Prostatitis
Benign Prostatic Hyperplasia
Carcinoma of the Prostate
Carcinoma of the Testis
Carcinoma of the Penis

Study Questions

The following questions are provided as a test for comprehension and as a study guide for use with the text chapters. Additional study material is located at http://health.jbpub.com/humandisease/, which contains useful eLearning tools such as an A&P review, animated flashcards, interactive online glossary, crossword puzzles, and Web links.

Key Terms

Define the following terms:

1. Seminoma _____

2. Prostate-specific antigen _____

Fill-in-the-Blank

1. The infectious agents that are the two main causes of acute urethritis acquired by sexual contact are

   _____ and _____. These infections are treated by _____.

2. Benign prostatic hyperplasia (BPH) is a common problem in older men. It produces symptoms of _____, resulting from compression of the _____ by the nodules of enlarged prostatic tissue.

3. There are many ways to treat BPH. The surgical procedure is called _____.

4. Prostatic epithelial cells secrete a protein called _____, which also can be detected in the bloodstream. Higher-than-normal levels are detected in the bloodstream of man with a disease called _____.

5. Testicular carcinomas are uncommon tumors. Many of these tumors produce a hormone called _____ and a protein antigen called _____.

6. Testicular malignant tumors that are composed of many different types of immature tissues are called

   _____.

7. Carcinoma of the penis is an uncommon tumor that almost never occurs in circumcised men. The agent responsible for the carcinoma is _____.

True/False

Tell whether each statement is true or false. If false, explain why the statement is incorrect.

1. Most prostate carcinomas arise from the inner group of prostatic glands surrounding the prostatic urethra. _____

   _____

2. Prostate-specific antigen is secreted by prostatic epithelial cells. _____

   _____

3. Most prostate carcinomas are very poorly differentiated, grow rapidly, and have a very poor prognosis. _____

   _____

Discussion Questions

1. What are the components of the male reproductive system? _____
   _____
   _____
   _____

2. What methods are available to detect carcinoma of the prostate? _____
   _____
   _____
   _____

3. How is carcinoma of the prostate treated? _____
   _____
   _____
   _____

4. Why do many physicians recommend conservative treatment of prostatic carcinoma in elderly men with well-
   differentiated tumors? _____
   _____
   _____
   _____

MALE REPRODUCTIVE SYSTEM

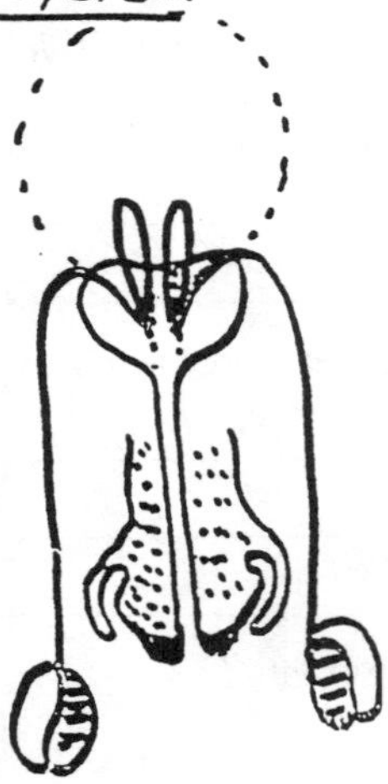

INFLAMMATION
   OF URETHRA
   OF PROSTATE
   OF EPIDIDYMIS

HYPERTROPHY
   OF PROSTATE
   (BPH)

NEOPLASMS
   OF PROSTATE
   - NATURAL HISTORY
   - EVALUATION·DIAGNOSIS
   OF TESTIS
   OF PENIS

PROSTATE CARCINOMA CONTROVERSIES
   SCREEN?
   TREAT?
        - WHY TREAT?
        - WHY NOT TREAT?

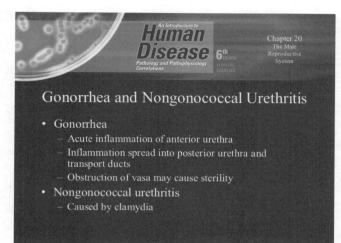

Gonorrhea and Nongonococcal Urethritis

- Gonorrhea
  - Acute inflammation of anterior urethra
  - Inflammation spread into posterior urethra and transport ducts
  - Obstruction of vasa may cause sterility
- Nongonococcal urethritis
  - Caused by clamydia

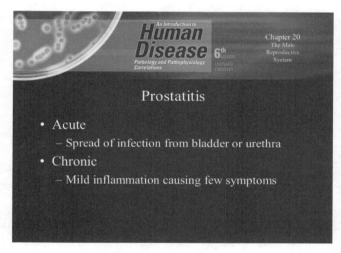

Prostatitis

- Acute
  - Spread of infection from bladder or urethra
- Chronic
  - Mild inflammation causing few symptoms

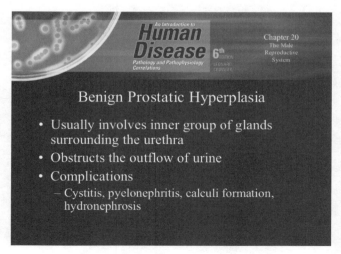

Benign Prostatic Hyperplasia

- Usually involves inner group of glands surrounding the urethra
- Obstructs the outflow of urine
- Complications
  - Cystitis, pyelonephritis, calculi formation, hydronephrosis

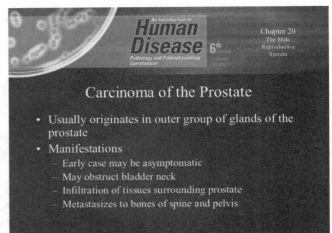

Carcinoma of the Prostate

- Usually originates in outer group of glands of the prostate
- Manifestations
  - Early case may be asymptomatic
  - May obstruct bladder neck
  - Infiltration of tissues surrounding prostate
  - Metastasizes to bones of spine and pelvis

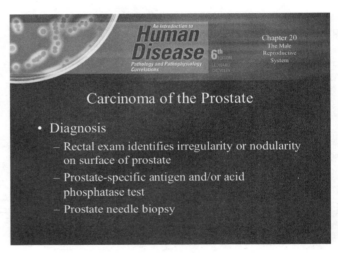

Carcinoma of the Prostate

- Diagnosis
  - Rectal exam identifies irregularity or nodularity on surface of prostate
  - Prostate-specific antigen and/or acid phosphatase test
  - Prostate needle biopsy

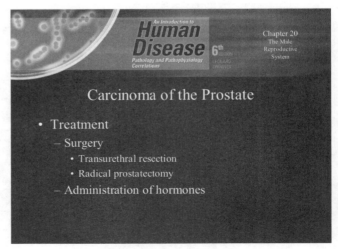

Carcinoma of the Prostate

- Treatment
  - Surgery
    - Transurethral resection
    - Radical prostatectomy
  - Administration of hormones

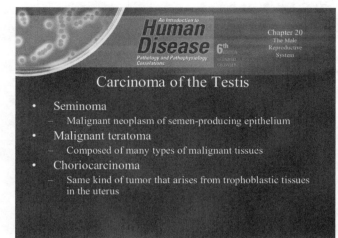

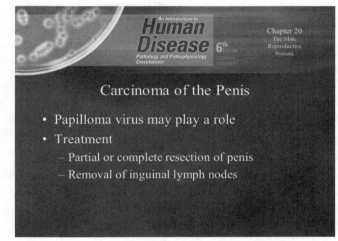

Chapter 21   The Liver and the Biliary System

Chapter Outline

The chapter outline provides you with an organizational guide to the topics and ideas presented in this chapter of the text.

Study Questions

The following questions are provided as a test for comprehension and as a study guide for use with the text chapters. Additional study material is located at http://health.jbpub.com/humandisease/, which contains useful eLearning tools such as an A&P review, animated flashcards, interactive online glossary, crossword puzzles, and Web links.

Key Terms

Define the following terms:

1. Hepatitis _____

2. Bilirubin _____

3. Bile _____

4. Jaundice _____

Fill-in-the-Blank

1. The iron-free pigment derived from breakdown of hemoglobin is called _____.

2. The substance present in bile that may precipitate within the bile to form gallstones is _____.

3. Some persons may have chronic hepatitis but show no symptoms of infection. This condition is called

   _____.

4. The antigen present in the blood of persons infected with hepatitis B is _____.

5. The most frequent cause of chronic hepatitis in the United States is _____.

6. Approximately _____ percent of persons infected with HCV are unable to eliminate the virus and become chronic carriers of the virus.

7. Persons with chronic hepatitis are at risk of two major complications, which are _____ and

   _____.

8. The two most common causes of cirrhosis are _____ and _____.

9. Two common causes of obstructive biliary cirrhosis are _____ and _____.

10. A child with a viral infection and a fever is given acetaminophen (Tylenol) rather than aspirin to control the fever to avoid the risk of a liver and central nervous system disease called _____.

11. Most gallstones are composed of _____.

True/False

Tell whether each statement is true or false. If false, explain why the statement is incorrect.

1. The infectious particle in the blood of persons with HBV infection is hepatitis B surface antigen. _____

   _____

2. Most HCV-infected persons are unable to eradicate the virus and become chronic carriers of the virus. _____

   _____

3. Many HCV-infected persons are asymptomatic. _____
_____

4. Chronic HCV infection is caused by ingestion of virus-contaminated food or water. _____
_____

5. Primary biliary cirrhosis is caused by chronic HCV infection. _____
_____

6. Primary biliary cirrhosis is an autoimmune disease in which the autoantibody is directed against bile duct epithelial cells. _____
_____

7. Secondary biliary cirrhosis is caused by longstanding obstruction of large extrahepatic bile ducts. _____
_____

8. Persons with cystic fibrosis of the pancreas have a normal life expectancy if the disease is treated by pancreatic enzymes and antibiotics. _____
_____

Identify

1. Construct a table comparing the major features of the three main types of hepatitis. (*Hint:* See Table 21-1.)

Characteristic	Hepatitis A	Hepatitis B	Hepatitis C

2. Alcoholic liver disease can be divided into three states of progressively increasing severity:

   a. _____

   b. _____

   c. _____

Discussion Questions

1. What are some of the main functions of the liver? _____
_____
_____
_____

2. How does the blood supply to the liver differ from the blood supply to other organs? _____
_____
_____
_____

3. Why does severe liver disease cause disturbances in blood clotting? _____

_____

_____

_____

4. What is the difference between hemoglobin and bilirubin? How does conjugated bilirubin differ from

unconjugated bilirubin? _____

_____

_____

_____

5. What is the difference between bilirubin and bile? What role does bile play in digestion? _____

_____

_____

_____

6. Describe the major structural changes and physiological derangements in patients with cirrhosis. What conditions

are associated with cirrhosis? _____

_____

_____

_____

7. Why is the pressure in the portal vein elevated in patients with cirrhosis? _____

_____

_____

_____

8. Why do patients with cirrhosis often accumulate fluid within their peritoneal cavity, which is called ascites?

_____

_____

_____

9. Why do patients with cirrhosis often develop varicose veins in their esophagus? _____

_____

_____

_____

10. In patients with cirrhosis, laboratory tests that measure the amounts of proteins concerned with the coagulation of the blood are frequently abnormal. Why? _____

_____

_____

_____

11. What is jaundice? How is jaundice classified? Under what circumstances do gallstones cause jaundice? _____

_____

_____

_____

12. What is hepatitis B virus (HBV) infection? How is it transmitted? What populations are at risk? How can it be prevented? _____

_____

_____

_____

13. What is fatty liver? With what other conditions is it associated? _____

_____

_____

_____

14. What is cholelithiasis? With what other conditions is it associated? _____

_____

_____

_____

15. What conditions may lead to hepatic cirrhosis? _____

_____

_____

_____

LIVER LOBULE

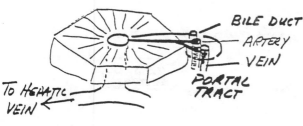

BILE DUCT
ARTERY
VEIN
PORTAL TRACT

TO HEPATIC VEIN

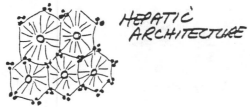

HEPATIC ARCHITECTURE

PORTAL CIRCULATION
HEPATIC BLOOD FLOW

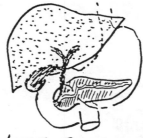

LIVER FUNCTIONS

1. METABOLISM
2. SYNTHESIS
3. DETOXIFICATION
4. STORAGE
5. EXCRETION

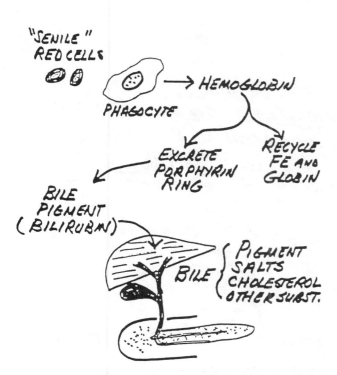

"SENILE" RED CELLS

PHAGOCYTE → HEMOGLOBIN

EXCRETE PORPHYRIN RING

RECYCLE FE AND GLOBIN

BILE PIGMENT (BILIRUBIN)

BILE { PIGMENT SALTS CHOLESTEROL OTHER SUBST.

HEPATITIS C : A BIG PROBLEM

• MOST HCV INFECTED PERSONS CAN'T ELIMINATE VIRUS
• COMMON CAUSE OF CHRONIC HEPATITIS NO PREVENTION AVAILABLE IF EXPOSED
• NO IMMUNIZING AGENT AVAILABLE
• MOST INFECTIONS ASYMPTOMATIC

WHO SHOULD BE CHECKED FOR HCV

• IV DRUG USERS
• PERSONS WHO RECEIVED AHG BEFORE 1987 OR BLOOD TRANSFUSION BEFORE 1992
• HEALTH CARE WORKERS EXPOSED TO BLOOD OR BODY FLUIDS
• "SEX INDUSTRY" WORKERS
• CHILDREN OF HCV INFECTED MOTHERS

WHAT IF PERSON INFECTED (ANTI- HCV)

• DOES PERSON HAVE CHRONIC HEPATITIS?
    ABNORMAL LIVER FUNCTION TESTS
    ABNORMAL LIVER BIOPSY
  TREAT PERSONS WITH CHRONIC HEPATITIS?
    INTERFERON
    RIBAVIRIN

COLLATERAL CIRCULATION PORTAL TO SYSTEMIC IN CIRRHOSIS

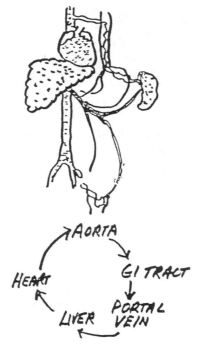

Aorta → GI TRACT → PORTAL VEIN → LIVER → Heart → Aorta

GALLSTONES

PATHOGENESIS
1. SUPERSATURATION OF BILE

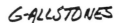

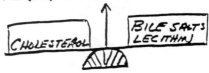

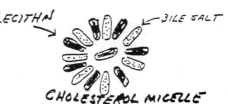

CHOLESTEROL MICELLE

2. INFECTION

COMPLICATIONS
DUCT OBSTRUCTION
- BILIARY COLIC
- JAUNDICE

CIRRHOSIS

RESULTING FROM HEPATOCYTE DAMAGE ("PORTAL CIRRHOSIS")
- ALCOHOLIC LIVER DISEASE
- CHRONIC HEPATITIS (HBV. HCV)
  SEVERE LIVER INJURY FROM DRUGS OR OTHER AGENTS
  VARIOUS GENETIC DISEASES
  HEMOCHROMATOSIS
  ALPHA, ANTITRYPSIN DEFICIENCY

RESULTING FROM BILE DUCT DAMAGE (BILIARY CIRRHOSIS)
- PRIMARY BILIARY CIRRHOSIS
  AUTOIMMUNE DISEASE
  DAMAGES SMALL INTRAHEPATIC DUCTS
- SECONDARY (OBSTRUCTIVE) BILIARY CIRRHOSIS
  CHRONIC OBSTRUCTION OF LARGE EXTRAHEPATIC BILE DUCTS

JAUNDICE
A MANIFESTATION NOT A DISEASE

CLASSIFICATION BY ETIOLOGY

HGB FROM RED CELL BREAKDOWN

RECYCE IRON AND GLOBIN

BILE PIGMENT

CONJUGATION. EXCRETION

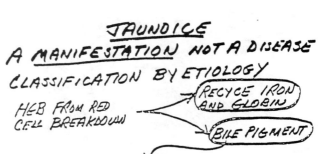

HEMOLYTIC   — BLOOD DESTRUCTION
HEPATOCELLULAR   — LIVER CELL DISEASE
OBSTRUCTIVE   — BILIARY OBSTRUCTION

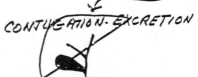

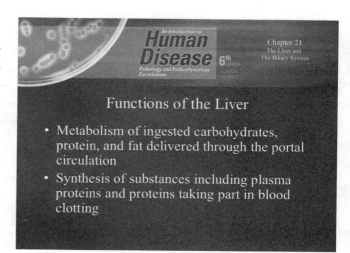

Functions of the Liver

- Metabolism of ingested carbohydrates, protein, and fat delivered through the portal circulation
- Synthesis of substances including plasma proteins and proteins taking part in blood clotting

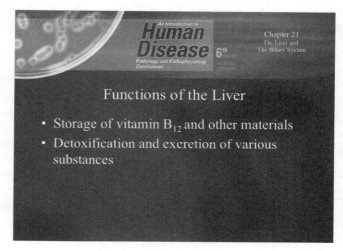

Functions of the Liver

- Storage of vitamin B_{12} and other materials
- Detoxification and excretion of various substances

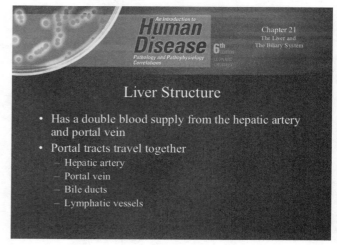

Liver Structure

- Has a double blood supply from the hepatic artery and portal vein
- Portal tracts travel together
  - Hepatic artery
  - Portal vein
  - Bile ducts
  - Lymphatic vessels

Notes

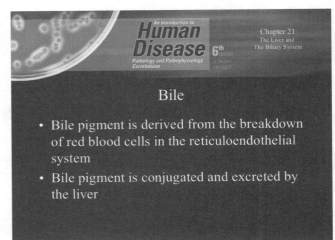

Bile

- Bile pigment is derived from the breakdown of red blood cells in the reticuloendothelial system
- Bile pigment is conjugated and excreted by the liver

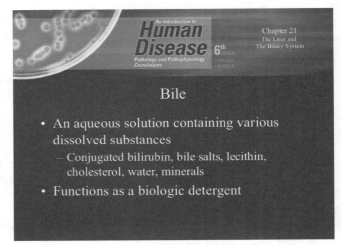

Bile

- An aqueous solution containing various dissolved substances
  - Conjugated bilirubin, bile salts, lecithin, cholesterol, water, minerals
- Functions as a biologic detergent

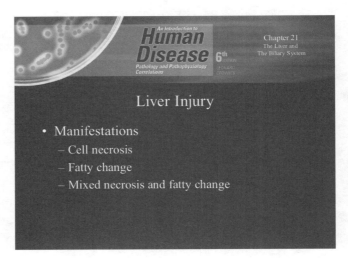

Liver Injury

- Manifestations
  - Cell necrosis
  - Fatty change
  - Mixed necrosis and fatty change

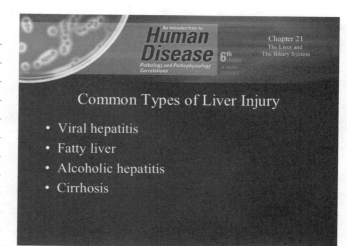

Common Types of Liver Injury

- Viral hepatitis
- Fatty liver
- Alcoholic hepatitis
- Cirrhosis

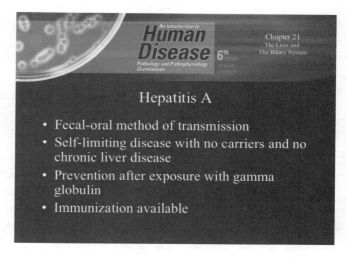

Hepatitis A

- Fecal-oral method of transmission
- Self-limiting disease with no carriers and no chronic liver disease
- Prevention after exposure with gamma globulin
- Immunization available

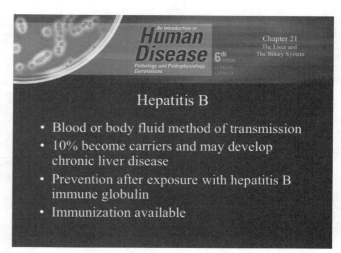

Hepatitis B

- Blood or body fluid method of transmission
- 10% become carriers and may develop chronic liver disease
- Prevention after exposure with hepatitis B immune globulin
- Immunization available

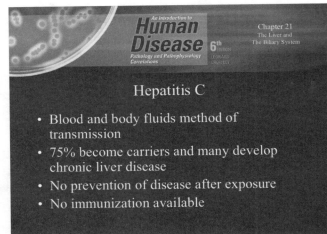

Hepatitis C

- Blood and body fluids method of transmission
- 75% become carriers and many develop chronic liver disease
- No prevention of disease after exposure
- No immunization available

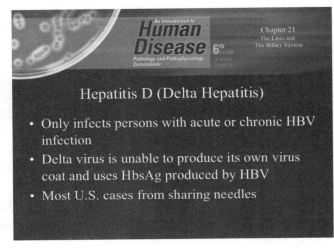

Hepatitis D (Delta Hepatitis)

- Only infects persons with acute or chronic HBV infection
- Delta virus is unable to produce its own virus coat and uses HbsAg produced by HBV
- Most U.S. cases from sharing needles

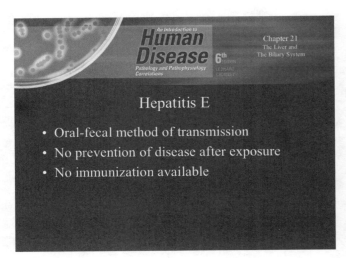

Hepatitis E

- Oral-fecal method of transmission
- No prevention of disease after exposure
- No immunization available

Notes

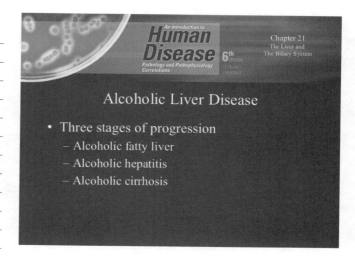

Alcoholic Liver Disease

- Three stages of progression
  - Alcoholic fatty liver
  - Alcoholic hepatitis
  - Alcoholic cirrhosis

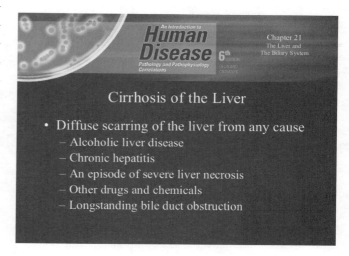

Cirrhosis of the Liver

- Diffuse scarring of the liver from any cause
  - Alcoholic liver disease
  - Chronic hepatitis
  - An episode of severe liver necrosis
  - Other drugs and chemicals
  - Longstanding bile duct obstruction

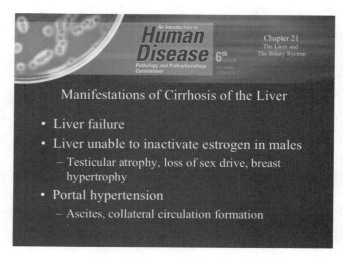

Manifestations of Cirrhosis of the Liver

- Liver failure
- Liver unable to inactivate estrogen in males
  - Testicular atrophy, loss of sex drive, breast hypertrophy
- Portal hypertension
  - Ascites, collateral circulation formation

Notes

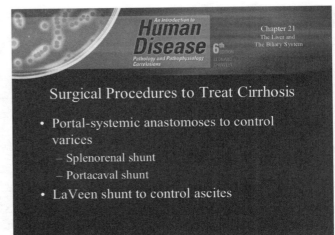

Surgical Procedures to Treat Cirrhosis

- Portal-systemic anastomoses to control varices
  - Splenorenal shunt
  - Portacaval shunt
- LaVeen shunt to control ascites

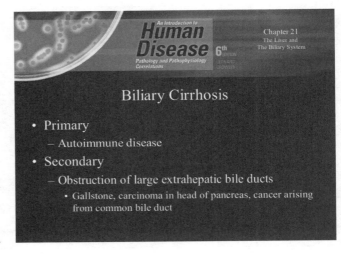

Biliary Cirrhosis

- Primary
  - Autoimmune disease
- Secondary
  - Obstruction of large extrahepatic bile ducts
    - Gallstone, carcinoma in head of pancreas, cancer arising from common bile duct

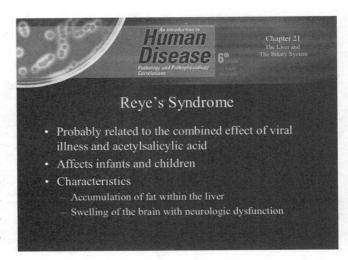

Reye's Syndrome

- Probably related to the combined effect of viral illness and acetylsalicylic acid
- Affects infants and children
- Characteristics
  - Accumulation of fat within the liver
  - Swelling of the brain with neurologic dysfunction

Notes

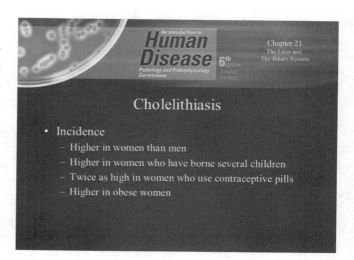

Chapter 21
The Liver and
The Biliary System

Cholelithiasis

- Incidence
  - Higher in women than men
  - Higher in women who have borne several children
  - Twice as high in women who use contraceptive pills
  - Higher in obese women

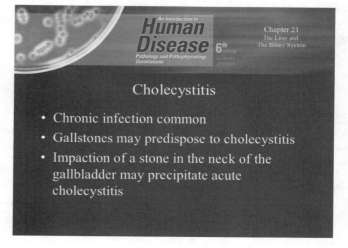

Chapter 21
The Liver and
The Biliary System

Cholecystitis

- Chronic infection common
- Gallstones may predispose to cholecystitis
- Impaction of a stone in the neck of the gallbladder may precipitate acute cholecystitis

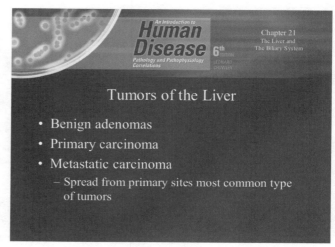

Chapter 21
The Liver and
The Biliary System

Tumors of the Liver

- Benign adenomas
- Primary carcinoma
- Metastatic carcinoma
  - Spread from primary sites most common type of tumors

Notes

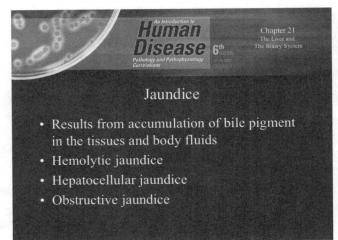

Chapter 21
The Liver and
The Biliary System

Jaundice

- Results from accumulation of bile pigment in the tissues and body fluids
- Hemolytic jaundice
- Hepatocellular jaundice
- Obstructive jaundice

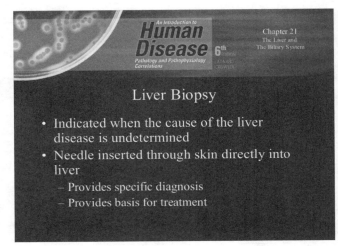

Chapter 21
The Liver and
The Biliary System

Liver Biopsy

- Indicated when the cause of the liver disease is undetermined
- Needle inserted through skin directly into liver
    - Provides specific diagnosis
    - Provides basis for treatment

Chapter Outline

The chapter outline provides you with an organizational guide to the topics and ideas presented in this chapter of the text.

Study Questions

The following questions are provided as a test for comprehension and as a study guide for use with the text chapters. Additional study material is located at http://health.jbpub.com/humandisease/, which contains useful eLearning tools such as an A&P review, animated flashcards, interactive online glossary, crossword puzzles, and Web links.

Key Terms

Define the following terms:

1. Ketone bodies _____

2. Ketosis _____

3. Diabetes _____

Fill-in-the-Blank

1. A blood test called _____ is often used to assess the average blood glucose level over the previous 6 to 12 weeks.

True/False

Tell whether the statement is true or false. If false, explain why the statement is incorrect.

1. Excess alcohol intake and gallstones are two factors that predispose a person to pancreatitis. _____

_____

Identify

1. Identify two factors that predispose a person to pancreatitis.

   a. _____

   b. _____

2. Construct a table comparing the major characteristics of the two major types of diabetes with respect to age of onset, body build, major complications, response to insulin, and response to oral antidiabetic drugs.

Characteristic Features	Type 1 Diabetes	Type 2 Diabetes

3. Identify six complications of poorly controlled diabetes.

   a. _____

   b. _____

   c. _____

   d. _____

e. _____

f. _____

Discussion Questions

1. Describe the major abnormalities in the pancreas of persons with cystic fibrosis of the pancreas. _____

   _____

   _____

   _____

2. Describe the major abnormalities in the lungs of persons with cystic fibrosis of the pancreas. _____

   _____

   _____

   _____

3. What are ketone bodies, and why are they elevated in persons with poorly controlled type 1 diabetes? _____

   _____

   _____

   _____

4. Why do some persons with type 2 diabetes develop diabetic coma even though they do not have ketosis? _____

   _____

   _____

   _____

5. Explain whether each of the following descriptors applies to cystic fibrosis of the pancreas.

   a. Transmitted as mendelian dominant trait _____

      _____

   b. Red cells sickle under low oxygen tension _____

      _____

   c. Characterized by secretion of thin, watery mucus _____

      _____

   d. Pancreas secretes excessive digestive enzymes that may digest the pancreas _____

      _____

   e. Frequently complicated by symptoms of chronic pulmonary disease _____

      _____

6. A 27-year-old woman has insulin-dependent diabetes. What abnormalities would be expected in this condition?

   _____

   _____

   _____

PANCREAS

ENDOCRINE
   ISLET CELL TUMORS
   ISLET "DEFICIENCY"

EXOCRINE
   TUMORS
   PANCREATITIS
   CYSTIC FIBROSIS —
      CF GENE MUTATION (CHR 7)
      IMPAIRS TRANSPORT OF
      ELECTROLYTES - WATER →
      — THICK MUCUS
      — HIGH SWEAT ELECTROLYTES

DIABETES: TWO DISEASES

TYPE 1 (IDDM)
   AUTOIMMUNE ISLET CELL DESTRUCTION
   CERTAIN HLA D TYPES PREDISPOSE

TYPE 2 (NIDDM)
   VERY COMMON DISEASE - EST. 7% POPULATION
   MUCH HIGHER FREQUENCY IN SOME GROUPS
   STRONG HEREDITARY PREDISPOSITION

   TISSUES INSULIN RESISTANT
   PANCREAS INCREASES INSULIN OUTPUT
   IMPAIRED BETA CELL FUNCTION DUE TO
      EXCESSIVE DEMAND FOR INSULIN

TWO TREATMENTS

TYPE 1

SUPPLY
INSULIN

TYPE 2

IMPROVE RESPONSIVENESS
TO INSULIN
   WEIGHT REDUCTION
   EXERCISE
   DRUGS

INCREASE INSULIN
ENDOGENOUS: HYPOGLYCEMIC
              DRUGS
EXOGENOUS: SUPPLY MORE
              INSULIN

DIABETES

	TYPE 1	TYPE 2
AGE	YOUNG	OLDER
BUILD	NORMAL	OVERWEIGHT
INSULIN LEVEL	LOW/ABSENT	HIGH
RESPONSE TO INSULIN	NORMAL	REDUCED
COMPLICATIONS	KETOACIDOSIS	HYPEROSMOLAR COMA

LONG TERM EFFECTS

INCREASED SUSCEPTIBILITY TO INFECTION
INCREASED VASCULAR DISEASE
   LARGE ARTERIES: ATHEROSCLEROSIS
   ARTERIOLES: ARTERIOLOSCLEROSIS
      EYES BLINDNESS
      KIDNEYS RENAL FAILURE
NERVE DEGENERATION: NEURITIS
METABOLIC PROBLEMS
   KETOACIDOSIS (TYPE 1)
   HYPEROSMOLAR COMA (TYPE 2)

GLUCOSE: AN ANABOLIC HORMONE

PROMOTES GLUCOSE ENTRY INTO CELL AND
USE AS ENERGY SOURCE
PROMOTES CONVERSION OF EXCESS FOR
STORAGE: AS GLYCOGEN IN LIVER AND MUSCLE
         AS FAT IN FAT CELLS, OR IN LIVER
         CELLS WHICH IS TRANSPORTED TO FAT CELLS
PROMOTES AMINO ACID ENTRY INTO CELLS
AND USE FOR PROTEIN SYNTHESIS

GLUCOSE

USE IT NOW
ENERGY

STORE TO USE LATER
AS GLYCOGEN
AS FAT

INSULIN LOWERS BLOOD GLUCOSE
ALL OTHER HORMONES RAISE GLUCOSE BY
VARIOUS MECHANISMS (BREAK DOWN
GLYCOGEN, CONVERT AMINO ACIDS TO GLUCOSE,
USE OTHER ENERGY SOURCES AND SPARE
GLUCOSE)

GROWTH HORMONE   CORTISOL
THYROID HORMONE   EPINEPHRINE
GLUCAGON

Notes

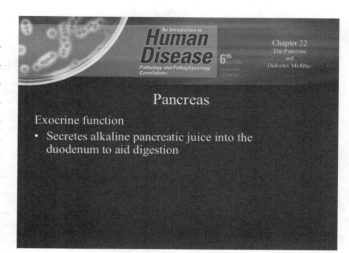

Pancreas

Exocrine function

- Secretes alkaline pancreatic juice into the duodenum to aid digestion

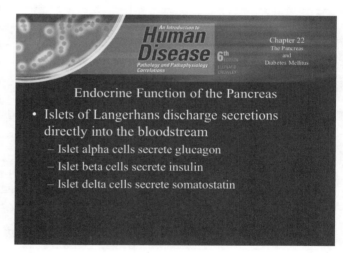

Endocrine Function of the Pancreas

- Islets of Langerhans discharge secretions directly into the bloodstream
  - Islet alpha cells secrete glucagon
  - Islet beta cells secrete insulin
  - Islet delta cells secrete somatostatin

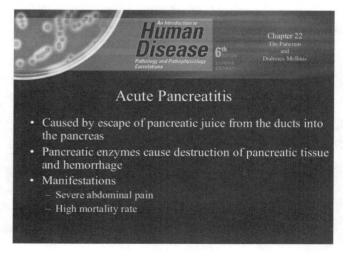

Acute Pancreatitis

- Caused by escape of pancreatic juice from the ducts into the pancreas
- Pancreatic enzymes cause destruction of pancreatic tissue and hemorrhage
- Manifestations
  - Severe abdominal pain
  - High mortality rate

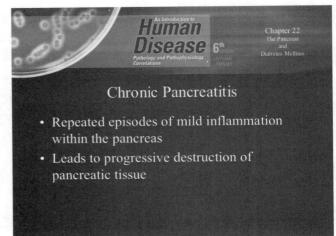

Chronic Pancreatitis

- Repeated episodes of mild inflammation within the pancreas
- Leads to progressive destruction of pancreatic tissue

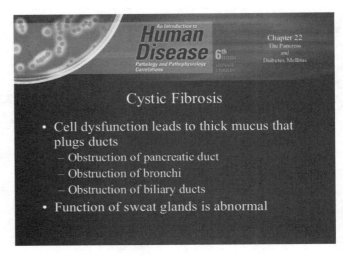

Cystic Fibrosis

- Cell dysfunction leads to thick mucus that plugs ducts
  - Obstruction of pancreatic duct
  - Obstruction of bronchi
  - Obstruction of biliary ducts
- Function of sweat glands is abnormal

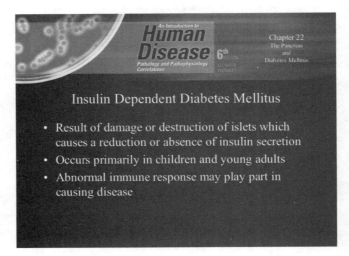

Insulin Dependent Diabetes Mellitus

- Result of damage or destruction of islets which causes a reduction or absence of insulin secretion
- Occurs primarily in children and young adults
- Abnormal immune response may play part in causing disease

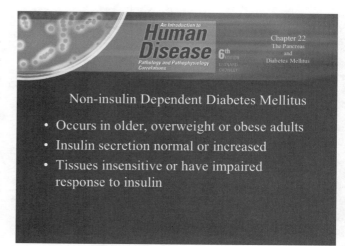

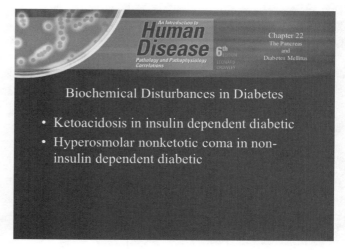

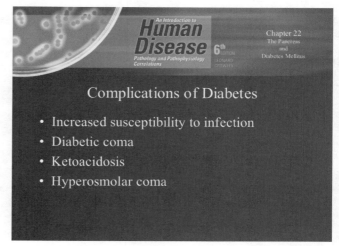

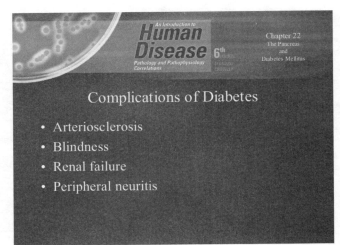

Complications of Diabetes

- Arteriosclerosis
- Blindness
- Renal failure
- Peripheral neuritis

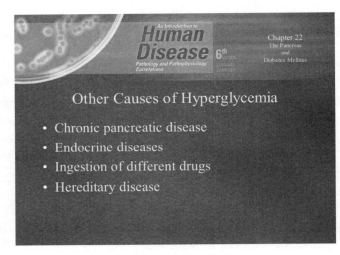

Other Causes of Hyperglycemia

- Chronic pancreatic disease
- Endocrine diseases
- Ingestion of different drugs
- Hereditary disease

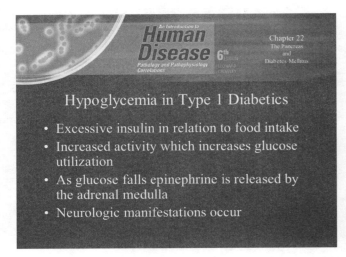

Hypoglycemia in Type 1 Diabetics

- Excessive insulin in relation to food intake
- Increased activity which increases glucose utilization
- As glucose falls epinephrine is released by the adrenal medulla
- Neurologic manifestations occur

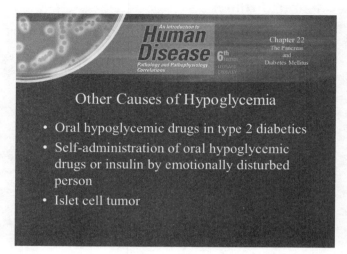

Other Causes of Hypoglycemia

- Oral hypoglycemic drugs in type 2 diabetics
- Self-administration of oral hypoglycemic drugs or insulin by emotionally disturbed person
- Islet cell tumor

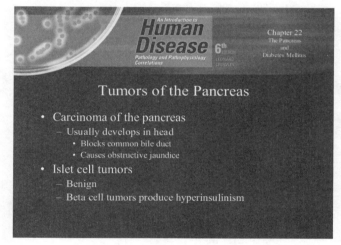

Tumors of the Pancreas

- Carcinoma of the pancreas
  - Usually develops in head
    - Blocks common bile duct
    - Causes obstructive jaundice
- Islet cell tumors
  - Benign
  - Beta cell tumors produce hyperinsulinism

Chapter Outline

The chapter outline provides you with an organizational guide to the topics and ideas presented in this chapter of the text.

Study Questions

The following questions are provided as a test for comprehension and as a study guide for use with the text chapters. Additional study material is located at http://health.jbpub.com/humandisease/, which contains useful eLearning tools such as an A&P review, animated flashcards, interactive online glossary, crossword puzzles, and Web links.

Key Terms

Define the following terms:

1. Reflux esophagitis _____

2. Barrett's esophagus _____

Fill-in-the-Blank

1. The inheritance of cleft lip and palate, which is related to interaction of multiple genes and environmental factors, is called a _____ inheritance pattern.

2. Each tooth is formed from a separate tooth bud, and _____ is deposited in the dentine and enamel as the tooth is formed.

3. To prevent staining of the teeth, the antibiotic _____ is not given to pregnant women or to children during the time when the teeth are forming.

4. Masses of bacteria intermixed with bacterial products and proteins from saliva form aggregates called _____ that adhere to the teeth and predispose a person to tooth decay.

5. The substance _____, when added to water supplies and toothpaste, helps prevent tooth decay.

6. Chronic gingivitis complicated by spread of the infection into the space between the teeth and gums to form pockets of pus is called _____.

7. A small superficial ulcer in the oral cavity is called _____.

8. Failure of the lower esophageal sphincter to open properly is called _____.

9. Inability of the lower esophageal sphincter to close properly is called _____. It leads to a condition called _____, which eventually may be complicated by a condition called _____.

10. The metaplastic change in the epithelium of the distal esophagus is called _____. It may predispose a person to the development of _____ in the distal esophagus.

11. An enzyme called _____ is required for the synthesis of prostaglandins, which have many functions. There are _____ forms of the enzyme.

12. Many cases of chronic gastritis appear to be caused by an organism called _____. This organism may also slightly increase the risk of developing two different types of gastric tumors, which are called _____ and _____.

13. If a person has a gastric or duodenal ulcer and is also colonized by an organism called _____, the person is treated not only with antacids but also with _____ to eradicate the organism.

True/False

Tell whether each statement is true or false. If false, explain why the statement is incorrect.

1. Many cases of acute gastritis are caused by nonsteroidal anti-inflammatory drugs (NSAIDs), which act by inhibiting an enzyme (cyclooxygenase) that is required to synthesize prostaglandins. _____

_____

2. There are two forms of cyclooxygenase (COX). One form (COX-1) promotes the synthesis of prostaglandins that protect the gastric mucosa from the harmful effects of gastric acid. The other form (COX-2) promotes the synthesis of prostaglandins that function as mediators of inflammation. _____

_____

Identify

1. Identify four harmful effects of obesity.

a. _____

b. _____

c. _____

d. _____

Matching

Match the abnormalities in the right column with the diseases in the left column.

Disease or Condition

1. ____ Regional enteritis (Crohn's disease)
2. ____ Meckel's diverticulitis
3. ____ Mesenteric artery thrombosis
4. ____ Chronic ulcerative colitis
5. ____ Antibiotic-associated colitis
6. ____ Non-tropical sprue
7. ____ Lactose intolerance
8. ____ Irritable bowel syndrome
9. ____ Colon diverticulosis
10. ____ Colon diverticulitis
11. ____ Intussusception
12. ____ Colon volvulus

Abnormality

A. Protrusion of mucosa through weak area in bowel wall

B. Hypersensitivity to wheat protein (gluten)

C. Inflammation of colon diverticula

D. Inflammation and ulceration of colon mucosa

E. Chronic inflammation and scarring of distal ileum

F. Deficiency of lactase enzyme

G. Overgrowth of *Clostridium difficile*

H. Inflammation of congenital small bowel diverticulum

I. Disturbed bowel function without structural changes

J. Rotary twist of sigmoid colon on its mesentery

K. Telescoping of proximal colon into distal colon

L. Extensive necrosis of small bowel and proximal colon

Discussion Questions

1. What are some of the major causes of esophageal obstruction? What symptoms does esophageal obstruction produce?

_____

_____

_____

2. How does acute appendicitis usually develop? What is the pathogenesis of acute appendicitis? _____

_____

_____

_____

3. What is intestinal obstruction? What symptoms does it produce? What are some of the common causes of intestinal obstruction? _____

_____

_____

_____

4. What symptoms and physical findings are likely to be encountered in a patient with a carcinoma of the colon? Why?

_____

_____

_____

5. One form of the cyclooxygenase enzyme (COX-1) promotes the synthesis of the prostaglandins that help protect the gastric mucosa from the potentially harmful effects of the acidic gastric juice. The other form of the enzyme (COX-2) promotes the synthesis of the prostaglandins that promote inflammation. If you wanted to take a nonsteroidal anti-inflammatory drug for an inflammatory disease such as arthritis but wanted to avoid the medication's side effects on the gastric mucosa, which of the COX enzymes would you want to inhibit? _____

_____

_____

_____

6. What conditions may cause intestinal obstruction? _____

_____

_____

_____

7. What conditions predispose a person to chronic diverticulosis of colon? _____

_____

_____

_____

8. As a result of the tumor, what conditions might be encountered in a patient with a small ulcerated carcinoma of the cecum? _____

_____

_____

_____

9. What condition usually results from a complete thrombosis or embolic occlusion of the superior mesenteric artery?

_____

_____

_____

PROBLEMS IN THE ORAL CAVITY AND ADJACENT TISSUES (LYMPH NODES AND SALIVARY GLANDS)

ORAL: INFLAMMATORY
   NON SPECIFIC: STOMATITIS
             ' GINGIVITIS
   SPECIFIC: CANKER SORE
            CANDIDA
            HERPES
            CHANCRE

CYSTS AND TUMORS
     PAPILLOMAS
     CYSTS
     "LEUKOPLAKIA"
     SQUAMOUS CELL CARCINOMA

PEPTIC ULCER

ACID
HELICOBACTER

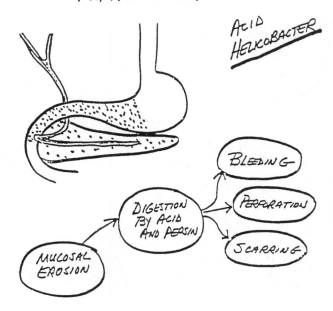

HEAD AND NECK MASSES

ENLARGED SALIVARY GLANDS
     INFLAMMATORY - OBSTRUCTING
                   CALCULI
     TUMORS

ENLARGED LYMPH NODES
     LYMPHOMAS - METASTATIC CANCER
     INFLAMMATIONS

ESOPHAGUS

SPHINCTER PROBLEMS
  — CARDIOSPASM
  — INCOMPETENT SPHINCTER
       REFLUX
       BARRETT'S ESOPHAGUS
MUCOSAL TEARS
NEOPLASMS.

ANTIBIOTIC ASSOCIATED COLITIS
- MANY PEOPLE CARRY CLOSTRIDIUM DIFFICILE IN THEIR COLON
- BROAD SPECTRUM ANTIBIOTIC DESTROYS INTESTINAL BACTERIA
- ANTIBIOTIC RESISTANT CLOSTRIDIUM NO LONGER HELD IN CHECK
- ORGANISM PRODUCES TOXINS THAT CAUSE INFLAMMATION - NECROSIS OF COLONIC MUCOSA
- CRAMPS AND BLOODY DIARRHEA

APPENDICITIS

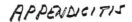

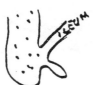 CECUM

INTRALUMINAL PRESSURE 0

INTRALUMINAL PRESSURE RISING

 MUCOSAL NECROSIS SPREAD OF INFLAMMATION

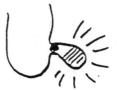

ORAL CAVITY

SMALL BOWEL

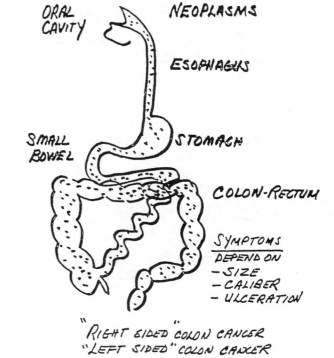

NEOPLASMS

ESOPHAGUS

STOMACH

COLON-RECTUM

SYMPTOMS
DEPEND ON
- SIZE
- CALIBER
- ULCERATION

"RIGHT SIDED" COLON CANCER
"LEFT SIDED" COLON CANCER

DIVERTICULA (SING. DIVERTICULUM)

SMALL BOWEL

CONGENITAL

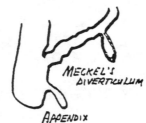

MECKEL'S DIVERTICULUM

APPENDIX

LINING MAY NOT BE THE SAME AS SMALL BOWEL MUCOSA.

COLON

ACQUIRED

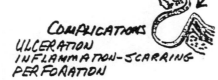

COMPLICATIONS
ULCERATION
INFLAMMATION-SCARRING
PERFORATION

HERNIA
  UNCOMPLICATED
  INCARCERATED
  STRANGULATED

VOLVULUS

INTUSSOSCEPTION

BANDS / ADHESIONS

NEOPLASMS

INTESTINAL OBSTRUCTION
  HIGH
  LOW

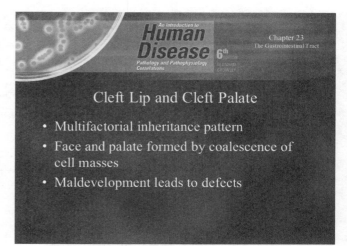

Chapter 23
The Gastrointestinal Tract

Cleft Lip and Cleft Palate

- Multifactorial inheritance pattern
- Face and palate formed by coalescence of cell masses
- Maldevelopment leads to defects

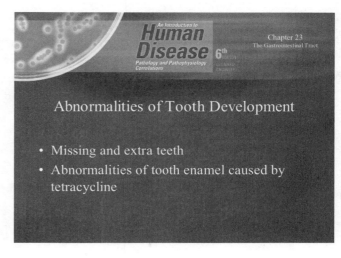

Chapter 23
The Gastrointestinal Tract

Abnormalities of Tooth Development

- Missing and extra teeth
- Abnormalities of tooth enamel caused by tetracycline

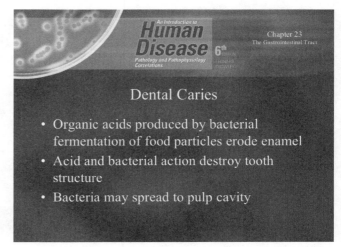

Chapter 23
The Gastrointestinal Tract

Dental Caries

- Organic acids produced by bacterial fermentation of food particles erode enamel
- Acid and bacterial action destroy tooth structure
- Bacteria may spread to pulp cavity

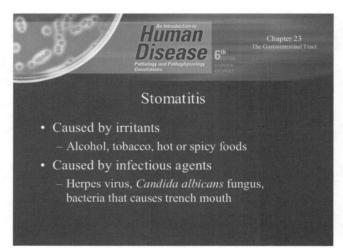

Stomatitis

- Caused by irritants
  - Alcohol, tobacco, hot or spicy foods
- Caused by infectious agents
  - Herpes virus, *Candida albicans* fungus, bacteria that causes trench mouth

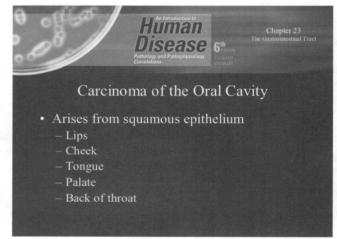

Carcinoma of the Oral Cavity

- Arises from squamous epithelium
  - Lips
  - Cheek
  - Tongue
  - Palate
  - Back of throat

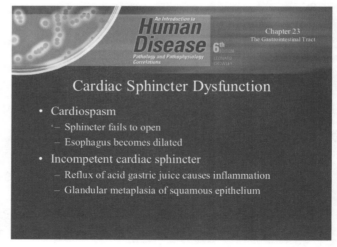

Cardiac Sphincter Dysfunction

- Cardiospasm
  - Sphincter fails to open
  - Esophagus becomes dilated
- Incompetent cardiac sphincter
  - Reflux of acid gastric juice causes inflammation
  - Glandular metaplasia of squamous epithelium

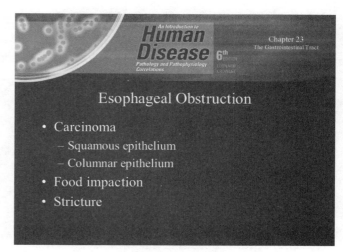

Esophageal Obstruction

- Carcinoma
  - Squamous epithelium
  - Columnar epithelium
- Food impaction
- Stricture

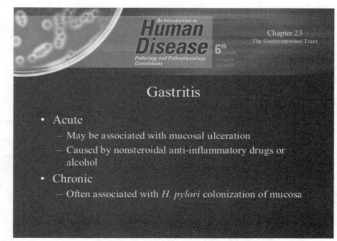

Gastritis

- Acute
  - May be associated with mucosal ulceration
  - Caused by nonsteroidal anti-inflammatory drugs or alcohol
- Chronic
  - Often associated with *H. pylori* colonization of mucosa

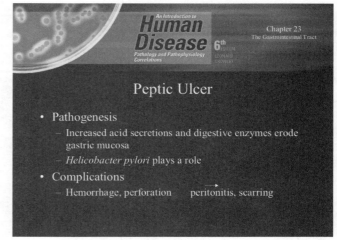

Peptic Ulcer

- Pathogenesis
  - Increased acid secretions and digestive enzymes erode gastric mucosa
  - *Helicobacter pylori* plays a role
- Complications
  - Hemorrhage, perforation → peritonitis, scarring

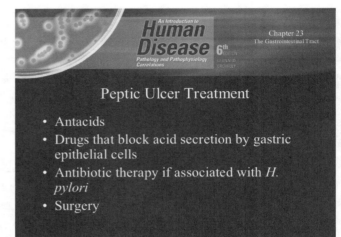

Peptic Ulcer Treatment

- Antacids
- Drugs that block acid secretion by gastric epithelial cells
- Antibiotic therapy if associated with *H. pylori*
- Surgery

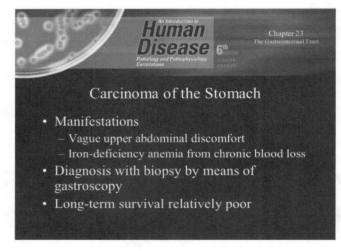

Carcinoma of the Stomach

- Manifestations
  - Vague upper abdominal discomfort
  - Iron-deficiency anemia from chronic blood loss
- Diagnosis with biopsy by means of gastroscopy
- Long-term survival relatively poor

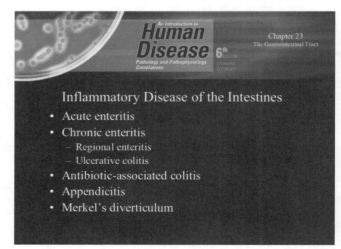

Inflammatory Disease of the Intestines

- Acute enteritis
- Chronic enteritis
  - Regional enteritis
  - Ulcerative colitis
- Antibiotic-associated colitis
- Appendicitis
- Merkel's diverticulum

Notes

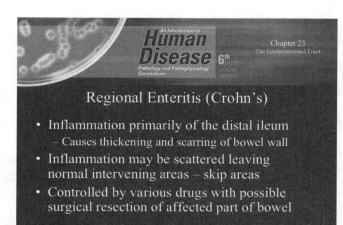

Regional Enteritis (Crohn's)

- Inflammation primarily of the distal ileum
  - Causes thickening and scarring of bowel wall
- Inflammation may be scattered leaving normal intervening areas – skip areas
- Controlled by various drugs with possible surgical resection of affected part of bowel

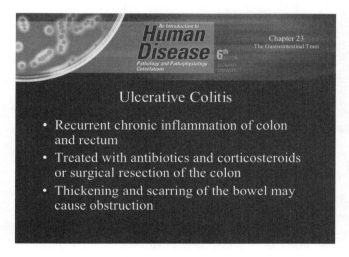

Ulcerative Colitis

- Recurrent chronic inflammation of colon and rectum
- Treated with antibiotics and corticosteroids or surgical resection of the colon
- Thickening and scarring of the bowel may cause obstruction

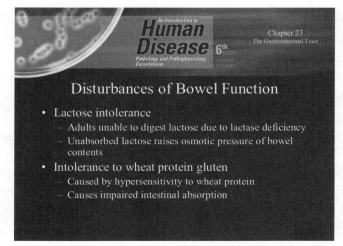

Disturbances of Bowel Function

- Lactose intolerance
  - Adults unable to digest lactose due to lactase deficiency
  - Unabsorbed lactose raises osmotic pressure of bowel contents
- Intolerance to wheat protein gluten
  - Caused by hypersensitivity to wheat protein
  - Causes impaired intestinal absorption

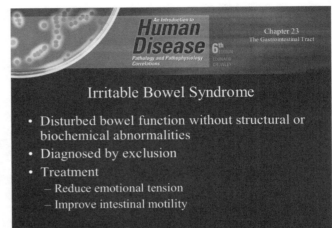

Irritable Bowel Syndrome

- Disturbed bowel function without structural or biochemical abnormalities
- Diagnosed by exclusion
- Treatment
  - Reduce emotional tension
  - Improve intestinal motility

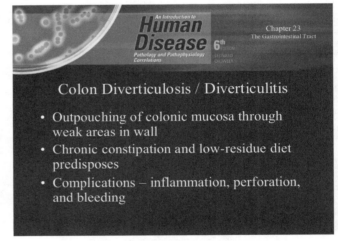

Colon Diverticulosis / Diverticulitis

- Outpouching of colonic mucosa through weak areas in wall
- Chronic constipation and low-residue diet predisposes
- Complications – inflammation, perforation, and bleeding

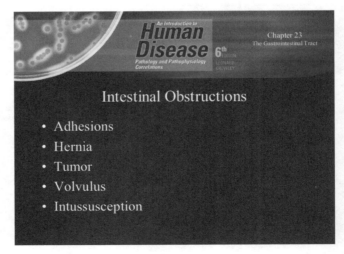

Intestinal Obstructions

- Adhesions
- Hernia
- Tumor
- Volvulus
- Intussusception

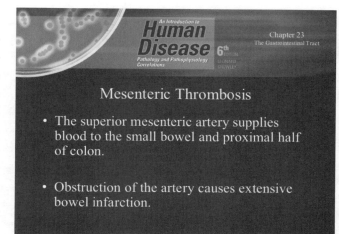

Mesenteric Thrombosis

- The superior mesenteric artery supplies blood to the small bowel and proximal half of colon.

- Obstruction of the artery causes extensive bowel infarction.

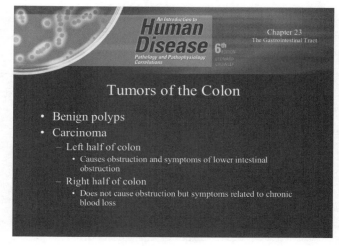

Tumors of the Colon

- Benign polyps
- Carcinoma
  - Left half of colon
    - Causes obstruction and symptoms of lower intestinal obstruction
  - Right half of colon
    - Does not cause obstruction but symptoms related to chronic blood loss

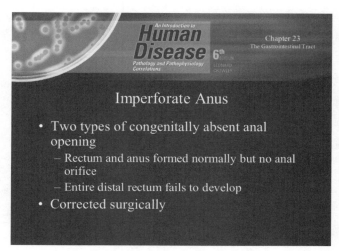

Imperforate Anus

- Two types of congenitally absent anal opening
  - Rectum and anus formed normally but no anal orifice
  - Entire distal rectum fails to develop
- Corrected surgically

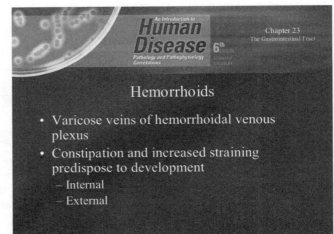

Hemorrhoids

- Varicose veins of hemorrhoidal venous plexus
- Constipation and increased straining predispose to development
  - Internal
  - External

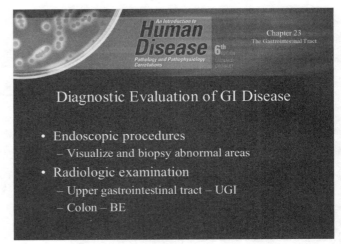

Diagnostic Evaluation of GI Disease

- Endoscopic procedures
  - Visualize and biopsy abnormal areas
- Radiologic examination
  - Upper gastrointestinal tract – UGI
  - Colon – BE

Chapter 24   Water, Electrolyte, and Acid-Base Balance

Chapter Outline

The chapter outline provides you with an organizational guide to the topics and ideas presented in this chapter of the text.

Body Water and Electrolytes
Interrelations of Intracellular and Extracellular Fluid
Units of Concentration of Electrolytes
Regulation of Body Fluid and Electrolyte Concentration
Disturbances of Water Balance
    Dehydration
    Overhydration
Disturbances of Electrolyte Balance
Acid–Base Balance
    Buffers
    Respiratory Control of Carbonic Acid
    Control of Bicarbonate Concentration
    Relation between pH and Ratio of Buffer Components
Disturbances of Acid–Base Balance
    Compensatory Mechanisms Responding to Disturbances in pH
    Metabolic Acidosis
    Respiratory Acidosis
    Metabolic Alkalosis
    Respiratory Alkalosis
    Diagnostic Evaluation of Acid–Base Balance

Study Questions

The following questions are provided as a test for comprehension and as a study guide for use with the text chapters. Additional study material is located at http://health.jbpub.com/humandisease/, which contains useful eLearning tools such as an A&P review, animated flashcards, interactive online glossary, crossword puzzles, and Web links.

Key Terms

Define the following terms:

1. Acidosis _____

2. Alkalosis _____

3. Electrolyte _____

4. pH _____

Fill-in-the-Blank

1. Positively charged ions are called _____, and negatively charged ions are called _____.

2. The units of concentration of electrolytes are expressed as _____.

3. The principal ions in intracellular fluids are _____.

Matching

The numbered column lists several clinical conditions associated with acid–base balance disturbances. The lettered column lists the four types of acid–base disturbances. Match the letter with the clinical condition. There are six conditions but only four acid–base disturbances, so some letters will be used more than once and some may not be used at all.

1. _____ Diabetes. Excessive ketone bodies formed.

2. _____ Hyperventilation. Fall in alveolar PCO_2 and blood carbonic acid.

3. _____ Impaired lung function caused by chronic pulmonary disease.

4. _____ Kidney failure. Retention of nonvolatile acids.

5. _____ Excess loss of gastric juice resulting from vomiting.

6. _____ Adrenal corticosteroid excess.

A. Metabolic acidosis

B. Respiratory acidosis

C. Metabolic alkalosis

D. Respiratory alkalosis

Discussion Questions

1. Body fluids are distributed within "compartments" as intracellular fluids and extracellular fluids. The extracellular fluids, in turn, are distributed between the fluid surrounding the cells (interstitial fluid) and that within the blood and lymph vessels (intravascular fluid). Which of these fluid compartments most closely resemble each other in

   electrolyte composition? _____

   _____

   _____

   _____

2. What percentage of body weight consists of water? _____
_____
_____
_____

3. What factors lead to overhydration of patients? _____
_____
_____
_____

4. What is the effect of prolonged use of diuretics on fluid and electrolyte balance? _____
_____
_____
_____

5. What is the source of the carbonic acid produced by the body? _____
_____
_____
_____

6. What is the source of the ketone bodies produced by the body? _____
_____
_____
_____

7. What is the source of the lactic acid produced by the body? _____
_____
_____
_____

8. What is the normal pH of blood and body fluids? _____
_____
_____
_____

9. What regulatory mechanisms does the body use to maintain the normal body fluid pH? _____
_____
_____
_____

10. How do blood buffers function to maintain normal body fluid pH? _____

_____

_____

_____

11. How do the lungs control the concentration of carbonic acid in the blood? _____

_____

_____

_____

12. How do the kidneys regulate the concentration of bicarbonate in the blood? _____

_____

_____

_____

13. What is the normal ratio of bicarbonate to carbonic acid at the normal pH of blood and body fluids? _____

_____

_____

_____

14. How does the body respond to a disease or condition characterized by an increase in carbonic acid in blood and

body fluids? _____

_____

_____

_____

15. How does the body respond when bicarbonate levels fall as a result of buffering of excess acids produced within

the body? _____

_____

_____

_____

16. What is metabolic acidosis? _____

_____

_____

_____

17. What are the principal causes of metabolic acidosis? _____

_____

_____

_____

18. What is respiratory alkalosis? _____

_____

_____

_____

19. What are the principal causes of respiratory alkalosis? _____

_____

_____

_____

20. What compensatory mechanisms does the body employ in an attempt to correct the pH change resulting from the
respiratory alkalosis? _____

_____

_____

_____

21. Why does excessive use of antacids disturb body pH? _____

_____

_____

_____

22. What effect do excess adrenal corticosteroids have on body pH? What mechanism is responsible for the
pH disturbance? What effect do the corticosteroids have on blood electrolytes? _____

_____

_____

_____

WATER · ELECTROLYTE INTAKE

LIQUIDS   1500 ml.
SOLIDS   700 ml.   ~ 2500 ml.
OXIDATION 250 ml

WATER · ELECTROLYTE LOSS

URINE   1000 - 1500 ml
STOOL   200
PERSPIRATION } 800   ~ 2500 ml.
WATER VAPOR }

DISTURBANCES

INADEQUATE   EXCESS

INADEQUATE INTAKE   OVERHYDRATION
EXCESSIVE LOSS
    : GI TRACT
    : URINE
    : PERSPIRATON

BODY WATER DISTRIBUTION

· 2/3 OF BODY WEIGHT IS WATER (ABOUT 10%
       LOWER IN ♂ BECAUSE OF HIGHER FAT CONTENT)
· 2/3 OF WATER IS INTRACELLULAR
○ 1/3 OF WATER IS EXTRACELLULAR
       AND MOST OF THIS IS INTERSTITIAL
       (BETWEEN CELLS). THE REST IS
       INTRAVASCULAR

ACID BASE BALANCE CONCEPTS

THE BODY GENERATES ACIDS
VOLATILE $CO_2 \rightarrow H_2CO_3$
NON VOLATILE
    METABOLIC: PHOSPHORIC   LACTIC
               SULFURIC   KETONE BODIES
               HYDROCHLORIC

BUT BODY FLUIDS ARE ALKALINE (pH ~ 7.4)

LUNGS EXCRETE CO_2

KIDNEYS EXCRETE NON VOLATILE ACIDS
       AND MAKE ALKALI (BICARBONATE)
BUFFERS MINIMIZE PH CHANGES

    BICARBONATE · CARBONIC ACID BUFFER
    · PHOSPHATES
    · PROTEINS

BUFFERS

MINIMIZE PH CHANGE

BICARBONATE   ⟶   PHOSPHATE
CARBONIC ACID   ⟵   HEMOGLOBIN
                          PROTEINS

STATUS OF BICARBONATE/CARBONIC ACID SYSTEM
REFLECTS STATUS OF ALL BUFFER SYSTEMS

PH DEPENDS ON RATIO OF COMPONENTS
NOT ABSOLUTE AMOUNTS

$$pH\ 7.4 : \frac{NAHCO_3}{H_2CO_3}, \frac{20}{1} : \frac{24\ mEq/l}{1.2\ mEq/l}$$

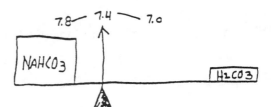

7.8 ⟋ 7.4 ⟍ 7.0

NAHCO₃   H₂CO₃

KIDNEYS   LUNGS
CONTROL   CONTROL
BICARBONATE   CARBONIC ACID
                    (pCO₂)

TOO MUCH: EXCRETE   CONTROL OF
          SOME   RESPIRATION
                         CONTROLS pCO₂
NOT ENOUGH: RECOVER
            ALL FILTERED
            MAKE MORE

KIDNEYS CONTROL BICARBONATE

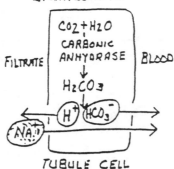

FILTRATE | $CO_2 + H_2O$ ↓ CARBONIC ANHYDRASE ↓ H_2CO_3 H^+ HCO_3^- | BLOOD
NA⁺

TUBULE CELL

"REABSORB" BICARBONATE
FORM MORE BICARBONATE

MECHANISM DEPENDS ON
EXCRETION OF H^+ IN
EXCHANGE FOR NA^+

EACH H^+ INTO FILTRATE
ALSO PRODUCES A HCO_3
WHICH IS ABSORBED
INTO BLOOD

LUNGS CONTROL CARBONIC ACID

ALVEOLAR
pCO₂
    ↓
CO₂ DISSOLVED
IN PLASMA
    ↓
H_2CO_3
    ↓
H^+ HCO_3

CONTROL OF
ALVEOLAR pCO₂
CONTROLS H_2CO_3

HYDROGEN ION (H^+) SECRETION BY TUBULE CELLS

$$H_2O + CO_2$$
CARBONIC ↓ ANHYDRASE
$$H_2CO_3$$

SECRETED INTO TUBULAR FILTRATE ← H^+ HCO_3 → ABSORBED INTO INTERSTITIAL FLUID AND THEN INTO BLOOD ALONG WITH Na^+ WHICH IS ABSORBED WHEN H^+ IS SECRETED

Na^+ →

FATE OF SECRETED H^+ IN FILTRATE

1. COMBINES WITH HCO_3^- IN FILTRATE
$$H^+ \cdot HCO_3 \longrightarrow H_2CO_3 \longrightarrow CO_2 + H_2O$$
["BICARBONATE REABSORPTION"]

2. COMBINES WITH AMMONIA (NH_3) SECRETED BY TUBULE CELLS AND EXCRETED AS NH_4^+

3. COMBINES WITH PHOSPHATE SALTS IN FILTRATE AND RELEASES Na^+ FOR ABSORPTION
[$Na_2HPO_4 + H^+ \longrightarrow NaH_2PO_4 + Na^+$]

EVERY H^+ SECRETED GENERATES A HCO_3^- WHICH IS ABSORBED WITH Na^+ AS $NAHCO_3$.
EVERY SECRETED H^+ YIELDS AN ABSORBED $NAHCO_3$.

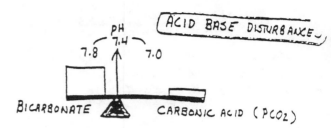

pH 7.4
7.8   7.0

BICARBONATE   CARBONIC ACID (PCO_2)

ACIDOSIS = EXCESS ACID OR INSUFFICIENT ALKALI
  METABOLIC = REDUCED BICARBONATE
  RESPIRATORY = INCREASED CARBONIC ACID

ALKALOSIS = EXCESS ALKALI OR INSUFFICIENT ACID
  METABOLIC = INCREASED BICARBONATE
  RESPIRATORY = REDUCED CARBONIC ACID

IF ONE COMPONENT OF RATIO DISTURBED THE BODY WILL
1. TRY TO ADJUST THE OTHER COMPONENT TO MAINTAIN RATIO, AND THEN
2. TRY TO RESTORE THE CONCENTRATION OF THE COMPONENT THAT WAS DISTURBED

---

pH RANGE
7.8 ——— 7.4 ——— 7.0

SODIUM BICARBONATE

AMOUNT OF SODIUM BICARBONATE LOST IN BUFFERING EXCESS ACID.

CARBONIC ACID

—Derangement of acid-base balance in metabolic acidosis.

DIABETIC KETOACIDOSIS
LACTIC ACIDOSIS
KIDNEY FAILURE

Derangement of acid-base balance in respiratory acidosis.

pH RANGE
7.8 ——— 7.4 ——— 7.0

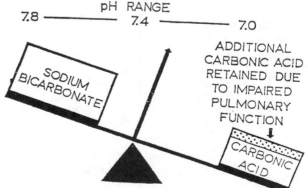

SODIUM BICARBONATE

ADDITIONAL CARBONIC ACID RETAINED DUE TO IMPAIRED PULMONARY FUNCTION

CARBONIC ACID

CHRONIC LUNG DISEASE LEADS TO ELEVATED PCO_2 AND CARBONIC ACID

METABOLIC ALKALOSIS
(EXCESS BICARBONATE)

1. LOSS OF GASTRIC ACID - ANTACIDS
2. CHLORIDE DEPLETION
3. CORTICOSTEROID EXCESS

① LOSS OF GASTRIC ACID - ANTACIDS

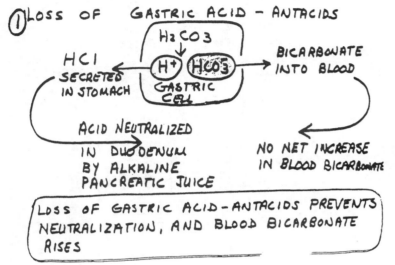

LOSS OF GASTRIC ACID - ANTACIDS PREVENTS NEUTRALIZATION, AND BLOOD BICARBONATE RISES

② CHLORIDE DEPLETION

NA AND CL ABSORBED TOGETHER IN PROXIMAL TUBULE

IF LESS CL, THEN LESS NA ABSORBED IN PROX. TUBULE

MORE NA IS ABSORBED IN DISTAL TUBULE IN EXCHANGE FOR $(K^+)(H^+)$ WHEN CHLORIDE DEPLETED

∴ MORE BICARBONATE FORMED IN EXCHANGE REACTION

③ STEROID EXCESS

CAUSES BOTH ALKALOSIS AND K^+ DEPLETION

STEROID PROMOTES NA^+ ABSORPTION FOR K^+ IN DISTAL TUBULE = POTASSIUM DEPLETION.

AS K^+ DEFICIENCY DEVELOPS, MORE NA^+ IS EXCHANGED FOR H^+

EACH H^+ SECRETED GENERATES HCO_3^- CONSERVED

COMPENSATION LIMITED
CAN'T HYPOVENTILATE (TO RAISE H_2CO_3)
CAN'T EXCRETE BICARBONATE
CORRECT POTASSIUM DEFICIENCY

RESPIRATORY ALKALOSIS

CAUSE: HYPERVENTILATION LOWERS PCO2
1. ANXIETY
2. DRUGS STIMULATE RESPIRATION
3. RESPIRATOR OVERVENTILATING PATIENT

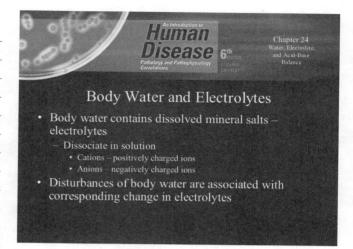

Body Water and Electrolytes

- Body water contains dissolved mineral salts –
  electrolytes
  - Dissociate in solution
    - Cations – positively charged ions
    - Anions – negatively charged ions
- Disturbances of body water are associated with
  corresponding change in electrolytes

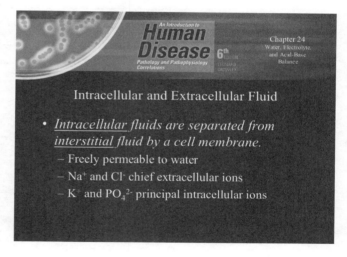

Intracellular and Extracellular Fluid

- *Intracellular fluids are separated from
  interstitial fluid by a cell membrane.*
  - Freely permeable to water
  - Na^+ and Cl^- chief extracellular ions
  - K^+ and PO_4^{2-} principal intracellular ions

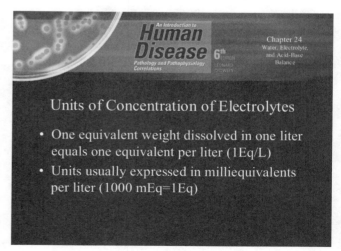

Units of Concentration of Electrolytes

- One equivalent weight dissolved in one liter
  equals one equivalent per liter (1Eq/L)
- Units usually expressed in milliequivalents
  per liter (1000 mEq=1Eq)

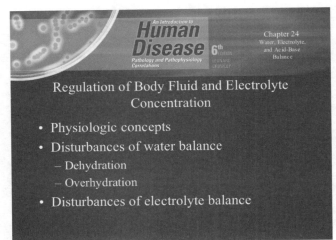

Regulation of Body Fluid and Electrolyte Concentration

- Physiologic concepts
- Disturbances of water balance
  - Dehydration
  - Overhydration
- Disturbances of electrolyte balance

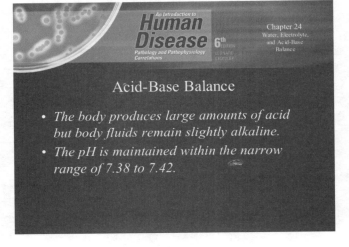

Acid-Base Balance

- *The body produces large amounts of acid but body fluids remain slightly alkaline.*
- *The pH is maintained within the narrow range of 7.38 to 7.42.*

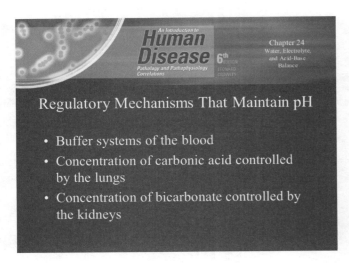

Regulatory Mechanisms That Maintain pH

- Buffer systems of the blood
- Concentration of carbonic acid controlled by the lungs
- Concentration of bicarbonate controlled by the kidneys

Notes

_____

_____

_____

_____

_____

_____

_____

_____

_____

_____

_____

_____

_____

_____

_____

_____

_____

_____

_____

_____

_____

_____

_____

_____

_____

_____

_____

_____

_____

_____

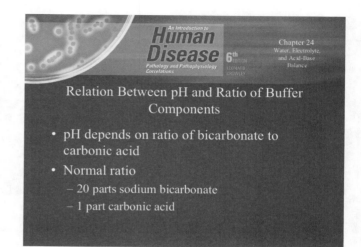

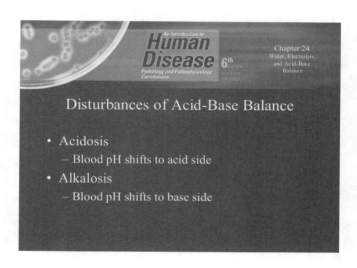

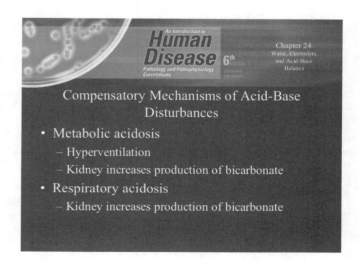

Water, Electrolyte, and Acid-Base Balance   287

Notes

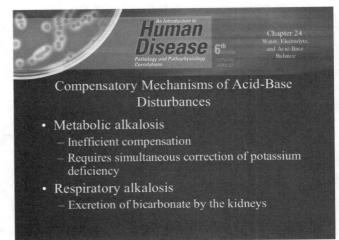

Chapter 24
Water, Electrolyte,
and Acid-Base
Balance

Compensatory Mechanisms of Acid-Base Disturbances

- Metabolic alkalosis
  - Inefficient compensation
  - Requires simultaneous correction of potassium deficiency
- Respiratory alkalosis
  - Excretion of bicarbonate by the kidneys

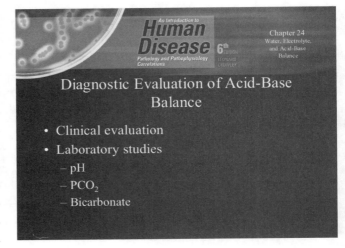

Chapter 24
Water, Electrolyte,
and Acid-Base
Balance

Diagnostic Evaluation of Acid-Base Balance

- Clinical evaluation
- Laboratory studies
  - pH
  - PCO_2
  - Bicarbonate

Chapter 25   The Endocrine Glands

Chapter Outline

The chapter outline provides you with an organizational guide to the topics and ideas presented in this chapter of the text.

Endocrine Functions and Dysfunctions
The Pituitary Gland
  Pituitary Hormones
  Physiologic Control of Pituitary Hormone Secretion
  Pituitary Hypofunction
  Overproduction of Growth Hormone
  Overproduction of Prolactin
The Thyroid Gland
  Actions of Thyroid Hormone
  Goiter
  Hypothyroidism
  Thyroiditis
  Tumors of the Thyroid
The Parathyroid Glands and Calcium Metabolism
  Hyperparathyroidism
  Hypoparathyroidism
The Adrenal Glands
  The Adrenal Cortex
  Disturbances of Adrenal Cortical Function
The Adrenal Medulla
  Tumors of the Adrenal Medulla
The Pancreatic Islets
The Gonads
Hormone Production by Nonendocrine Tumors
Stress and the Endocrine System
Obesity
  Causes of Obesity
  Health Consequences of Obesity
  Treatment of Obesity

Study Questions

The following questions are provided as a test for comprehension and as a study guide for use with the text chapters. Additional study material is located at http://health.jbpub.com/humandisease/, which contains useful eLearning tools such as an A&P review, animated flashcards, interactive online glossary, crossword puzzles, and Web links.

Key Terms

Define the following terms:

1. Acromegaly _____

2. Amenorrhea _____

3. Goiter _____

4. Cretinism _____

5. Thyroiditis _____

6. Pheochromocytoma _____

7. Myxedema _____

True/False

Tell whether the statement is true or false. If false, explain why the statement is incorrect.

1. Some NSAIDs have a more selective inhibitory effect on COX-2 than on COX-1, thereby suppressing the prostaglandins that cause inflammation in the tissues without significantly interfering with the synthesis of the prostaglandins that protect the gastric mucosa. _____

   _____

Identify

1. Identify five major complications of obesity.

   a. _____

   b. _____

   c. _____

   d. _____

   e. _____

Matching

Match the abnormalities in the right column with the diseases in the left column.

1. _____ Acromegaly
2. _____ Amenorrhea-galactorrhea syndrome
3. _____ Exophthalmic goiter
4. _____ Addison's disease
5. _____ Cushing's disease
6. _____ Cushing's syndrome
7. _____ Cretinism
8. _____ Chronic thyroiditis
9. _____ Hyperparathyroidism
10. _____ Hyperaldosteronism
11. _____ Pheochromocytoma
12. _____ Morbid obesity

A. Neonatal hypothyroidism
B. ACTH-producing pituitary tumor
C. Growth hormone-secreting pituitary tumor
D. Administration of excess adrenal corticosteroids
E. Autoantibody-induced thyroid hyperfunction
F. Autoantibody-induced destruction of adrenal cortex
G. Autoantibody-induced destruction of thyroid gland
H. Prolactin-secreting pituitary tumor
I. Hormone-secreting parathyroid tumor
J. Catecholamine-secreting adrenal tumor
K. Excess food intake
L. Aldosterone-secreting adrenal cortical tumor

Discussion Questions

1. What are the major hormones produced by the pituitary gland? What factors regulate secretion of pituitary hormones? (See Fig. 25-1.) _____

_____

_____

_____

2. What is the effect of overproduction of growth hormone? _____

_____

_____

_____

3. What factors regulate the rate of production of thyroid hormone? What are the major effects of an abnormal output of thyroid hormone? (See Table 25-1.) _____

_____

_____

_____

4. What is the difference between cretinism and myxedema? _____

_____

_____

_____

5. Why does the thyroid gland become enlarged in persons with a nontoxic goiter? _____

_____

_____

_____

6. What is the difference between thyroiditis and thyrotoxicosis? What are the roles played by autoantibodies in the pathogenesis of these diseases? _____

_____

_____

_____

7. What are the main classes of adrenal cortical hormones, and what are their functions? _____

_____

_____

_____

8. What diseases result from adrenal cortical dysfunction? _____

_____

_____

_____

9. How is parathyroid hormone output regulated? What are the possible effects of parathyroid dysfunction?

_____

_____

_____

10. Describe the "stomach stapling" procedures used to treat morbid obesity. _____

_____

_____

_____

11. A 27-year-old woman has small, diffuse toxic goiter. What manifestations would you expect in this patient?

_____

_____

_____

12. A 25-year-old woman has acromegaly. What manifestations would you expect in this patient? _____

_____

_____

_____

13. A 35-year-old woman has hypothyroidism due to chronic thyroiditis. What manifestations would you expect in this condition? _____

_____

_____

_____

14. A 64-year-old man has Addison's disease due to atrophy of both adrenal glands. What clinical manifestations would you expect in this condition? _____

_____

_____

_____

15. A 46-year-old woman has Cushing's disease due to hyperplasia of both adrenal glands. What are the manifestations that are often encountered in this condition? _____

_____

_____

_____

EXOCRINE = DUCT = DIGESTIVE
ENDOCRINE = NO DUCT = REGULATOR

DISORDERS
    OVERACTIVITY
    UNDERACTIVITY

FACTORS INFLUENCING CLINICAL EFFECTS
    AGE
    SEX
    DEGREE OF FUNCTIONAL DERANGEMENT

REGULATORY PATTERNS
   - CONTROLLED BY ANOTHER GLAND
   - CONTROLLED/REGULATED BY
     PRODUCT UNDER GLAND
     CONTROL
   - FEEDBACK INHIBITIONS

MAJOR PITUITARY HORMONES
ANTERIOR LOBE

NAME	ACTION
TSH (THYROTROPIN)	STIMULATES THYROID GROWTH AND SECRETION
ACTH (CORTICOTROPIN)	STIMULATES ADRENAL CORTEX GROWTH AND SECRETION
GROWTH HORMONE (SOMATOTROPIN)	PROMOTES GROWTH
FSH } GONADOTROPINS	STIMULATES FOLLICLE GROWTH / SPERMATOGENESIS
LH }	STIMULATES OVULATION LUTEINIZATION OF FOLLICLE / TESTOSTERONE SECRETION
PROLACTIN	MILK SECRETION

INTERMEDIATE LOBE

MSH (MELANOCYTE STIMULATING HORMONE)	STIMULATES MELANIN SYNTHESIS IN MELANOCYTES

POSTERIOR LOBE

ADH (ANTIDIURETIC HORMONE) ["WATER RETENTION HORMONE"]	PROMOTES WATER RETENTION BY KIDNEY
OXYTOCIN	CAUSES MILK EJECTION UTERINE CONTRACTION

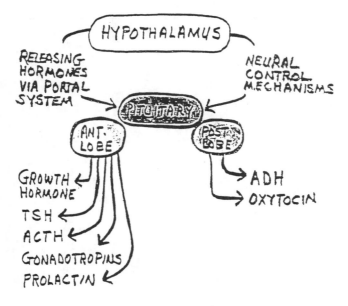

ANT. LOBE MALFUNCTIONS

GROWTH HORMONE:	GIGANTISM ACROMEGALY	DWARFISM
ACTH	CUSHING'S DISEASE	
PROLACTIN	AMENORRHEA GALACTORRHEA SYNDROME	

FEEDBACK CONTROL OF TROPIC HORMONES

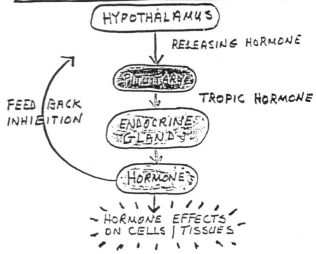

ESSENTIAL CONCEPTS

- HORMONE LEVEL CONTROLS IT OWN RELEASE VIA FEEDBACK INHIBITION

- HIGH HORMONE LEVEL SHUTS OFF "TROPIC HORMONE

- LOW HORMONE LEVEL (FROM ENDOCRINE-GLAND FAILURE) STIMULATES TROPIC HORMONE OUTPUT IN AN ATTEMPT TO INCREASE HORMONE LEVEL INTO NORMAL RANGE

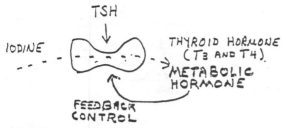

TSH

IODINE

THYROID HORMONE
(T3 AND T4)
METABOLIC
HORMONE

FEEDBACK
CONTROL

METABOLIC EFFECTS

CARDIOVASCULAR
NEUROMUSCULAR
EMOTIONAL- INTELLECTUAL
(GROWTH AND CNS DEVELOPMENT IN
NEWBORN)

SYNTHESIS - STORAGE - RELEASE

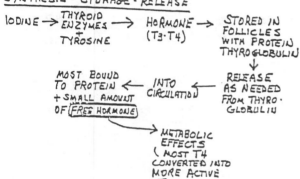

IODINE → THYROID ENZYMES + TYROSINE → HORMONE (T3·T4) → STORED IN FOLLICLES WITH PROTEIN THYROGLOBULIN

↓

MOST BOUND TO PROTEIN + SMALL AMOUNT OF FREE HORMONE ← INTO CIRCULATION ← RELEASE AS NEEDED FROM THYRO· GLOBULIN

↓

METABOLIC EFFECTS
(MOST T4 CONVERTED INTO MORE ACTIVE T3)

CLINICAL SYNDROMES

GRAVE'S DISEASE
(HYPERTHYROIDISM)
(THYROTOXICOSIS)

CRETINISM
MYXEDEMA

GOITER

ENLARGED THYROID

DECREASED FUNCTION
    CHRONIC THYROIDITIS
    CONGENITAL GOITER
NORMAL FUNCTION (UNDER DURESS)
    DIFFUSE (COLLOID) GOITER
    NODULAR GOITER
INCREASED FUNCTION
    GRAVES DISEASE

THYROID DYSFUNCTIONS

PERIODIC INCREASED NEED FOR HORMONE
(ADOLESCENCE, PREGNANCY)
GLAND ENLARGES TO INCREASE OUTPUT
AND SHRINKS WHEN INCREASED HORMONE
NEED SUBSIDES

ABNORMAL PROTEIN MADE BY LYMPHOID
CELLS ATTACH TO THYROID CELLS

TWO DIFFERENT EFFECTS DEPENDING ON
PROPERTIES OF ABNORMAL PROTEIN

- DESTROYS THYROID CELLS AND
  CAUSES THYROID HYPOFUNCTION
  (CHRONIC THYROIDITIS)
- OVERSTIMULATES THYROID CELLS AND
  CAUSES THYROID HYPERFUNCTION
  (HYPERTHYROIDISM)

IN NEWBORNS

FAILURE OF GLAND TO DEVELOP

GLAND FORMS BUT LACKS ENZYMES
NEEDED TO MAKE HORMONE

MOTHER INGESTED DRUG THAT
IMPAIRED NEONATAL·FETAL THYROID
FUNCTION

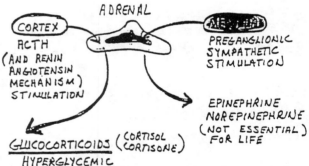

ADRENAL

CORTEX
ACTH
(AND RENIN
ANGIOTENSIN
MECHANISM)
STIMULATION

MEDULLA
PREGANGLIONIC
SYMPATHETIC
STIMULATION

EPINEPHRINE
NOREPINEPHRINE
(NOT ESSENTIAL)
FOR LIFE

GLUCOCORTICOIDS (CORTISOL CORTISONE)
HYPERGLYCEMIC
    DECREASE GLUCOSE UTILIZATION. USE FAT
    BREAK DOWN PROTEIN INTO AMINO ACIDS
    AND USE TO MAKE GLUCOSE
    (GLUCONEOGENESIS)
ANTI- INFLAMMATORY

MINERALOCORTICOIDS (ALDOSTERONE)

PROMOTES RETENTION OF SALT AND WATER
IN RESPONSE TO LOW SALT, WATER, BLOOD
    VOLUME, BLOOD PRESSURE
(RENIN· ANGIOTENSIN· ALDOSTERONE MECHANISM)

SEX HORMONES

MOSTLY ANDROGENS
PROMOTE SEX DRIVE

ADRENAL CORTICAL DISEASE

HYPOFUNCTION
ADDISONS DISEASE

HYPERFUNCTION

GLUCOCORTICOID EXCESS: CUSHING'S
- ACTH PRODUCING PITUITARY TUMOR
- ADMINISTRATION OF STEROIDS
- ADRENAL CORTICAL STEROID-PRODUCING TUMOR
- NON-ENDOCRINE MALIGNANT TUMOR PRODUCING STEROID-LIKE PROTEINS

MINERALOCORTICOID EXCESS: ALDOSTERONE PRODUCING TUMOR
- EXCESS NA+ REABSORPTION RAISES BLOOD SODIUM, BLOOD VOLUME, BLOOD PRESSURE
- EXCESS K+ EXCRETION LOWERS BLOOD POTASSIUM. MUSCLE WEAKNESS
- LOW PLASMA RENIN (NEGATIVE FEEDBACK EFFECT).

ADRENAL MALFUNCTION

	CORTEX: EXCESS	DEFICIENCY
GLUCOCORTICOIDS	HIGH GLUCOSE GIRDLE OBESITY STRIAE PROTEIN BREAKDOWN MUSCLE LOSS LOSS OF BONE DENSITY	LOW GLUCOSE
MINERALOCORTICOIDS	RETENTION OF SALT AND WATER BLOOD PRESSURE AND VOLUME RISE	LOSS OF SALT AND WATER BLOOD PRESSURE AND VOLUME FALL
SEX HORMONES	—	—
FEED BACK EFFECT	—	PIGMENTATION
CONDITION/DISEASE	CUSHING'S DISEASE	ADDISON'S DISEASE

	MEDULLA: EXCESS	DEFICIENCY
CATECHOLAMINES	HIGH BLOOD PRESSURE JITTERY ANXIOUS	—

Adrenal Medullary Hormones
SYNTHESIZED IN MEDULLA
STORED IN MEDULLA
RELEASED IN RESPONSE TO NERVE IMPULSES FROM ANS (PREGANGLIONIC SYMPATHETIC)

FUNCTIONING TUMORS OF ADRENAL MEDULLA RAISE BLOOD PRESSURE

PANCREATIC ISLETS
ALPHA CELLS (20%): GLUCAGON-RAISES GLUCOSE
BETA CELLS (70%): INSULIN- LOWERS GLUCOSE
MISC. OTHER CELL TYPES

STIMULUS FOR INSULIN RELEASE: RISE IN BLOOD GLUCOSE AFTER EATING

INSULIN: AN ANABOLIC HORMONE
PROMOTES GLUCOSE ENTRY INTO CELL AND USE AS ENERGY SOURCE
PROMOTES CONVERSION OF EXCESS FOR STORAGE
- AS GLYCOGEN IN LIVER AND MUSCLE
- AS FAT IN FAT CELLS, AND IN LIVER CELLS WHICH IS TRANSPORTED TO FAT CELLS
PROMOTES ENTRY OF AMINO ACIDS INTO CELLS AND PROTEIN SYNTHESIS

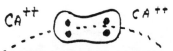

Ca^{++} — — — — — Ca^{++}

PARATHYROID GLANDS REGULATE
LEVEL OF IONIZED CALCIUM
- PROMOTE Ca^{++} UPTAKE
- PROMOTE MOBILIZATION FROM BONE
- PROMOTE P EXCRETION (AND CA
    RETENTION) BY KIDNEYS.
(ANTAGONIZED BY CALCITONIN)

HYPERFUNCTION   HYPOFUNCTION

ADENOMA   SURGICAL REMOVAL

PANCREATIC
ISLETS

ISLET   DIABETES
CELL
TUMOR

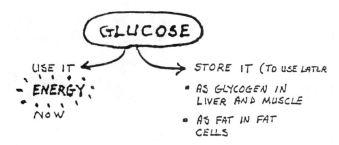

GLUCOSE

USE IT   STORE IT (TO USE LATER
- ENERGY -   • AS GLYCOGEN IN
NOW   LIVER AND MUSCLE
                 • AS FAT IN FAT
                   CELLS

HORMONES AND BLOOD GLUCOSE

INSULIN: PROMOTES GLUCOSE ENTRY INTO
        CELL AND USE AS ENERGY SOURCE
        AND STORAGE OF EXCESS
        LOWERS BLOOD GLUCOSE

ALL OTHER METABOLIC HORMONES RAISE
BLOOD GLUCOSE BY VARIOUS MECHANISMS
   • BREAKING DOWN GLYCOGEN (RAPID RESPONSE)
   • MAKING NEW GLUCOSE FROM PROTEIN BREAKDOWN
   • CONSERVING GLUCOSE BY USING OTHER
       ENERGY SOURCES INSTEAD OF GLUCOSE

	GLYCOGEN BREAKDOWN	GLUCONEO GENESIS	OTHER ENERGY SOURCES
GROWTH HORMONE		⊕	⊕
THYROID	+		
GLUCAGON	+		
CORTISOL		⊕	⊕
EPINEPHRINE	+		

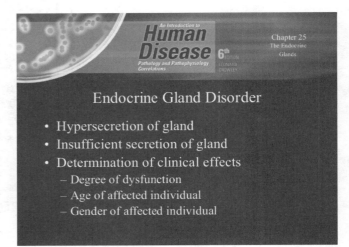

Endocrine Gland Disorder

- Hypersecretion of gland
- Insufficient secretion of gland
- Determination of clinical effects
  - Degree of dysfunction
  - Age of affected individual
  - Gender of affected individual

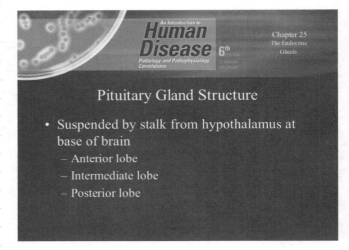

Pituitary Gland Structure

- Suspended by stalk from hypothalamus at base of brain
  - Anterior lobe
  - Intermediate lobe
  - Posterior lobe

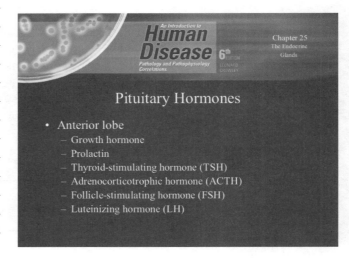

Pituitary Hormones

- Anterior lobe
  - Growth hormone
  - Prolactin
  - Thyroid-stimulating hormone (TSH)
  - Adrenocorticotrophic hormone (ACTH)
  - Follicle-stimulating hormone (FSH)
  - Luteinizing hormone (LH)

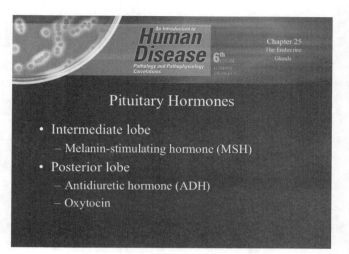

Pituitary Hormones

- Intermediate lobe
  - Melanin-stimulating hormone (MSH)
- Posterior lobe
  - Antidiuretic hormone (ADH)
  - Oxytocin

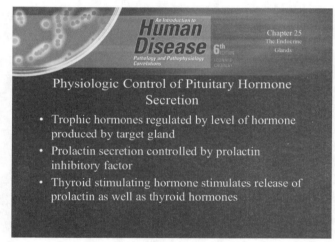

Physiologic Control of Pituitary Hormone Secretion

- Trophic hormones regulated by level of hormone produced by target gland
- Prolactin secretion controlled by prolactin inhibitory factor
- Thyroid stimulating hormone stimulates release of prolactin as well as thyroid hormones

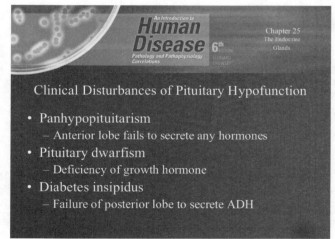

Clinical Disturbances of Pituitary Hypofunction

- Panhypopituitarism
  - Anterior lobe fails to secrete any hormones
- Pituitary dwarfism
  - Deficiency of growth hormone
- Diabetes insipidus
  - Failure of posterior lobe to secrete ADH

Notes

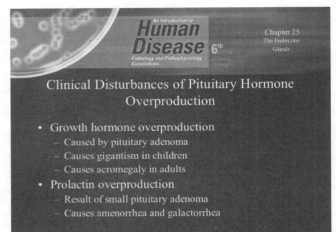

Clinical Disturbances of Pituitary Hormone Overproduction

- Growth hormone overproduction
  - Caused by pituitary adenoma
  - Causes gigantism in children
  - Causes acromegaly in adults
- Prolactin overproduction
  - Result of small pituitary adenoma
  - Causes amenorrhea and galactorrhea

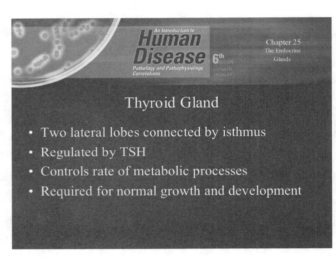

Thyroid Gland

- Two lateral lobes connected by isthmus
- Regulated by TSH
- Controls rate of metabolic processes
- Required for normal growth and development

Hyperthyroidism	Hypothyroidism
Rapid pulse	Slow pulse
Increased metabolism	Decreased metabolism
Hyperactive reflexes	Sluggish reflexes
Emotional lability	Placid and phlegmatic
GI effect – diarrhea	GI effect - constipation
Warm, moist skin	Cold, dry skin

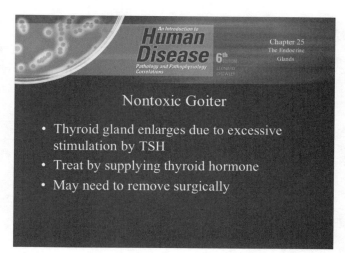

Nontoxic Goiter

- Thyroid gland enlarges due to excessive stimulation by TSH
- Treat by supplying thyroid hormone
- May need to remove surgically

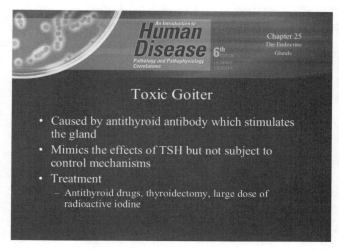

Toxic Goiter

- Caused by antithyroid antibody which stimulates the gland
- Mimics the effects of TSH but not subject to control mechanisms
- Treatment
  - Antithyroid drugs, thyroidectomy, large dose of radioactive iodine

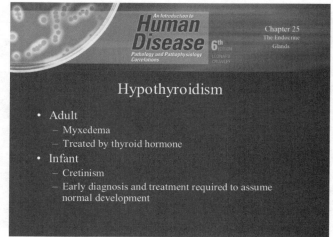

Hypothyroidism

- Adult
  - Myxedema
  - Treated by thyroid hormone
- Infant
  - Cretinism
  - Early diagnosis and treatment required to assume normal development

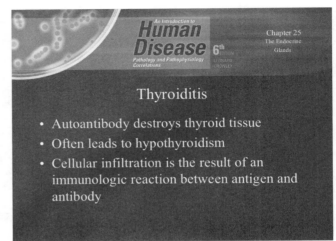

Thyroiditis

- Autoantibody destroys thyroid tissue
- Often leads to hypothyroidism
- Cellular infiltration is the result of an immunologic reaction between antigen and antibody

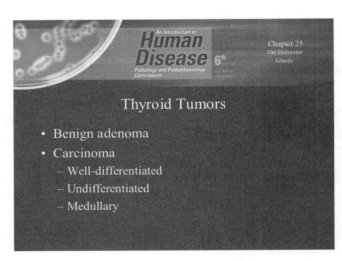

Thyroid Tumors

- Benign adenoma
- Carcinoma
  - Well-differentiated
  - Undifferentiated
  - Medullary

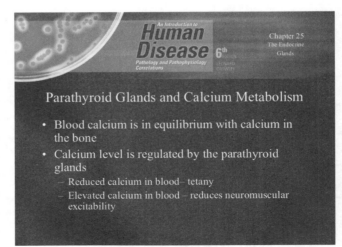

Parathyroid Glands and Calcium Metabolism

- Blood calcium is in equilibrium with calcium in the bone
- Calcium level is regulated by the parathyroid glands
  - Reduced calcium in blood– tetany
  - Elevated calcium in blood – reduces neuromuscular excitability

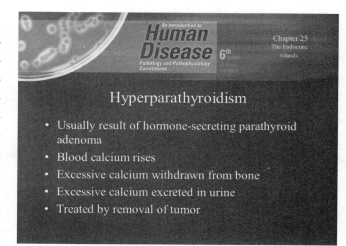

Hyperparathyroidism

- Usually result of hormone-secreting parathyroid adenoma
- Blood calcium rises
- Excessive calcium withdrawn from bone
- Excessive calcium excreted in urine
- Treated by removal of tumor

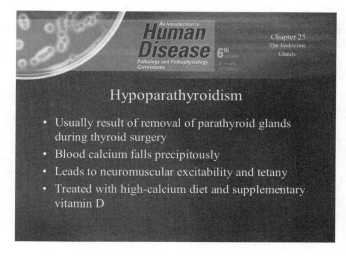

Hypoparathyroidism

- Usually result of removal of parathyroid glands during thyroid surgery
- Blood calcium falls precipitously
- Leads to neuromuscular excitability and tetany
- Treated with high-calcium diet and supplementary vitamin D

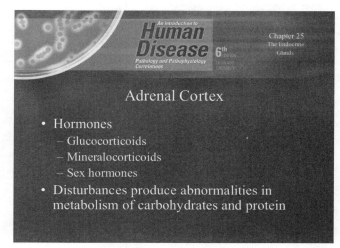

Adrenal Cortex

- Hormones
  - Glucocorticoids
  - Mineralocorticoids
  - Sex hormones
- Disturbances produce abnormalities in metabolism of carbohydrates and protein

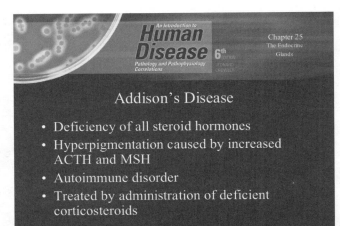

Addison's Disease

- Deficiency of all steroid hormones
- Hyperpigmentation caused by increased ACTH and MSH
- Autoimmune disorder
- Treated by administration of deficient corticosteroids

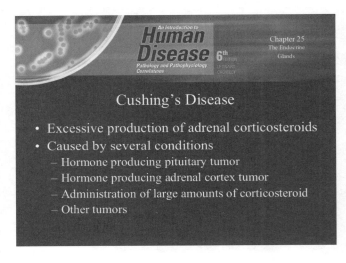

Cushing's Disease

- Excessive production of adrenal corticosteroids
- Caused by several conditions
  - Hormone producing pituitary tumor
  - Hormone producing adrenal cortex tumor
  - Administration of large amounts of corticosteroid
  - Other tumors

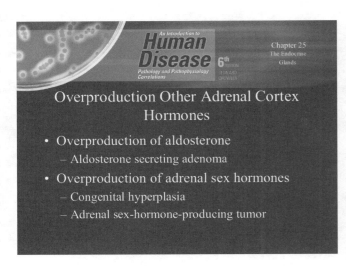

Overproduction Other Adrenal Cortex Hormones

- Overproduction of aldosterone
  - Aldosterone secreting adenoma
- Overproduction of adrenal sex hormones
  - Congenital hyperplasia
  - Adrenal sex-hormone-producing tumor

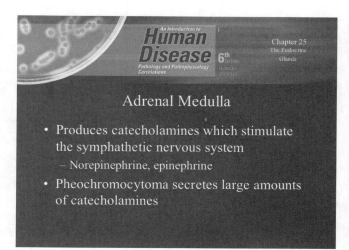

Adrenal Medulla

- Produces catecholamines which stimulate the symphathetic nervous system
  – Norepinephrine, epinephrine
- Pheochromocytoma secretes large amounts of catecholamines

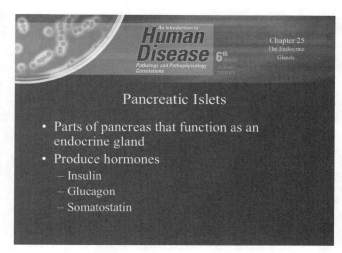

Pancreatic Islets

- Parts of pancreas that function as an endocrine gland
- Produce hormones
  – Insulin
  – Glucagon
  – Somatostatin

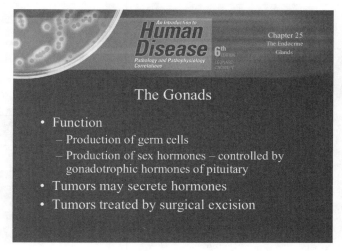

The Gonads

- Function
  – Production of germ cells
  – Production of sex hormones – controlled by gonadotrophic hormones of pituitary
- Tumors may secrete hormones
- Tumors treated by surgical excision

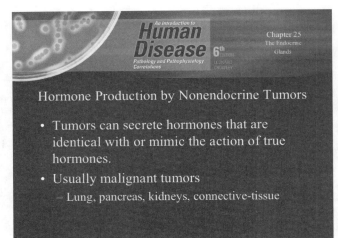

Hormone Production by Nonendocrine Tumors

- Tumors can secrete hormones that are identical with or mimic the action of true hormones.
- Usually malignant tumors
  - Lung, pancreas, kidneys, connective-tissue

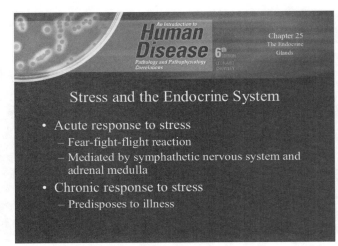

Stress and the Endocrine System

- Acute response to stress
  - Fear-fight-flight reaction
  - Mediated by symphathetic nervous system and adrenal medulla
- Chronic response to stress
  - Predisposes to illness

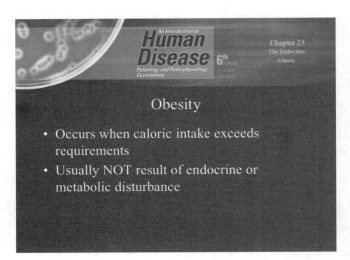

Obesity

- Occurs when caloric intake exceeds requirements
- Usually NOT result of endocrine or metabolic disturbance

Chapter 26   The Nervous System

Chapter Outline

The chapter outline provides you with an organizational guide to the topics and ideas presented in this chapter of the text.

Structure and Function
Development of the Nervous System
Muscle Tone and Voluntary Muscle Contraction
Muscle Paralysis
    Flaccid Paralysis
    Spastic Paralysis
Cerebral Injury
Neural Tube Defects
    Anencephaly
    Spina Bifida
    Prenatal Detection of Neural Tube Defects
Hydrocephalus
Stroke
    Cerebral Thrombosis
    Stroke Caused by Arteriosclerosis of Extracranial Arteries
    Cerebral Hemorrhage
    Manifestations of Stroke
    Rehabilitation of the Stroke Patient
Transient Ischemic Attack
Cerebral Aneurysm
Infections of the Nervous System
    Meningitis Caused by Bacteria and Fungi
    Viral Infections
Creutzfeldt-Jakob Disease
    Mad Cow Disease
Alzheimer's Disease
Multiple Sclerosis
Parkinson's Disease
Degenerative Diseases of Motor Neurons
Tumors of the Nervous System
    Tumors of the Peripheral Nerves
    Tumors of the Brain
    Tumors of the Spinal Cord
Peripheral Nerve Disorders
    Peripheral Nerve Injury
    Polyneuritis (Peripheral Neuritis)
    Guillain Barré Syndrome (Idiopathic Polyneuritis)
Neurologic Manifestations of Human Immunodeficiency Virus Infections
    AIDS Virus Infections of the Nervous System
    Opportunistic Infections of the Nervous System
    AIDS-Related Tumors

Study Questions

The following questions are provided as a test for comprehension and as a study guide for use with the text chapters. Additional study material is located at http://health.jbpub.com/humandisease/, which contains useful eLearning tools such as an A&P review, animated flashcards, interactive online glossary, crossword puzzles, and Web links.

Key Terms

Define the following terms:

1. Upper motor neuron lesion _____

2. Lower motor neuron lesion _____

3. Parkinson's disease _____

4. Meningitis _____

5. Stroke _____

6. Anencephaly _____

Fill-in-the-Blank

1. The frequency of neural tube defects can be reduced significantly by ingestion of the vitamin _____ before conception and during pregnancy.

2. Failure of the cephalic end of the neural tube to close leads to a condition called _____, and failure of the cephalic end to close properly leads to a condition called _____.

3. A stroke is a vascular injury to the brain that is classified as either an _____ or a _____.

4. A sac-like protrusion of the lining of a cerebral artery through a defect or weak area in the arterial wall is called a _____. The major complication of this condition is _____, and the treatment of this complication is _____.

5. A brief, temporary episode of neurologic dysfunction, followed by return of normal cerebral functions, is called a _____.

6. Recent onset of marked atrophy and weakness of skeletal muscles that were previously affected by poliomyelitis many years previously but were followed by complete recovery is called _____.

7. Creutzfeldt-Jakob disease is caused by an abnormal form of a protein called a _____. The disease may result either from a spontaneous mutation of a normal gene that codes for a normal protein or from _____.

8. This type of abnormal protein causes a disease in cows called _____, which can be transmitted to humans by _____.

9. A hereditary disease characterized by formation of multiple tumors arising from peripheral nerves is called _____.

10. Multiple sclerosis plaques within the brain can be demonstrated by a procedure called _____.

11. A poorly differentiated astrocytic tumor arising in older adults is called a _____.

12. A malignant brain tumor arising from the cerebellum in children is called a _____.

13. A brain tumor arising from the cerebral meninges is called a _____, and a brain tumor arising from the ependymal lining of the ventricular system is called an _____.

14. Persons with an immunodeficiency disease called _____ are prone to develop lymphomas of the nervous system that respond poorly to treatment.

True/False

Tell whether each statement is true or false. If false, explain why the statement is incorrect.

1. Post-polio syndrome is characterized by late onset of muscle atrophy, weakness, and fatigue many years after recovery from poliomyelitis. _____

   _____

2. The abnormal form of the prion protein is identical to the normal form except for the configuration of the abnormal protein (the way the protein is folded). _____

   _____

3. Mad cow disease is a type of rabies that causes cows to become aggressive and hostile. _____

   _____

4. New-variant Creutzfeldt-Jakob disease is acquired by eating meat from cows infected with abnormal prions.

   _____

Identify

1. What are the two principal types of neural tube defects?

   a. _____

   b. _____

2. Identify three neurologic manifestations of HIV infection.

   a. _____

   b. _____

   c. _____

Discussion Questions

1. Briefly describe the organization of the central nervous system. Describe the function and circulation of cerebrospinal fluid. _____

   _____

   _____

   _____

2. Describe how flaccid paralysis differs from spastic paralysis. _____

   _____

   _____

   _____

3. List or describe possible harmful effects of a severe blow to the head. _____
_____
_____
_____

4. Explain how atherosclerosis of a carotid artery can cause a stroke. _____
_____
_____

5. What are the common causes of hydrocephalus? How does a brain tumor cause hydrocephalus? _____
_____
_____

6. List and describe briefly the methods available to detect a neural tube defect in a fetus. _____
_____
_____

7. Describe the two types of shunt procedures used to treat hydrocephalus, distinguishing between them with respect
to the site of drainage from the shunt. _____
_____
_____

8. What is a brief episode of neurologic dysfunction that subsides spontaneously in a short time? _____
_____
_____

9. What are the effects of hydrocephalus in a middle-aged adult? _____
_____
_____

10. What is a congenital aneurysm of the circle of Willis? _____
_____
_____

ORGANIZATION OF THE NERVOUS SYSTEM

CENTRAL
CEREBRUM
CEREBELLUM
BRAIN STEM / CORD

PERIPHERAL
NERVES
GANGLIA

- MENINGES
- VESSELS
- VENTRICULAR SYSTEM
  CHOROID PLEXUSES
- NEURONS / GLIA
- CROSSED PATHWAYS
- CRANIAL CAVITY

DEGENERATIVE DISEASES

MULTIPLE SCLEROSIS

MYELIN
SHEATH
DAMAGE
↓
GLIAL
SCARS

ALZHEIMERS DISEASE

NEURON
DEGENERATION
↓
- NEUROFIBRILLARY
  TANGLES
- PLAQUES
- AMYLOID

"LITTLE STROKES"

MULTIFOCAL
SMALL
CVAs

PRION DISEASE

OCCURS IN PEOPLE AND ANIMALS
TRANSMITTED BY PRION CONTAMINATED
    BODY TISSUES
CAUSES RAPID NEUROLOGIC DETERIORATION

CLASSIC CJ DISEASE

MAD COW DISEASE

IN UK TRACED TO CATTLE FEED
FORTIFIED WITH PROTEIN TISSUES
FROM PRION INFECTED SHEEP.

NEW VARIANT CJ DISEASE

? EATING MEAT FROM INFECTED COWS
NO CASES DESCRIBED IN US

HYDROCEPHALUS

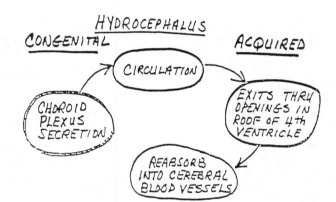

CONGENITAL ——— ACQUIRED

CIRCULATION

CHOROID
PLEXUS
SECRETION

EXITS THRU
OPENINGS IN
ROOF OF 4th
VENTRICLE

REABSORB
INTO CEREBRAL
BLOOD VESSELS

VASCULAR LESIONS

STROKES
    ISCHEMIC = PLUGGED VESSEL

     HEMORRHAGIC = RUPTURED VESSEL

TIA
    ACUTE ISCHEMIA - FLOW RE-ESTABLISHED
    NO RESIDUAL DAMAGE

CAROTID PLAQUES

    SOURCE OF THROMBO-EMBOLIC
    MATERIAL
    ?MANAGEMENT

CONGENITAL CEREBRAL ANEURYSMS

   - DEFECT CONGENITAL
   - PROTRUSION ACQUIRED

INFECTIONS

ENCEPHALITIS		MENINGITIS
VIRAL	BACTERIAL	OTHERS
HERPES	MENINGOCOCCUS	FUNGI
ARBOVIRUS	PNEUMOCOCCUS	PROTOZOA
	H. INFLUENZA	

TUMORS

PRIMARY   METASTATIC

MENINGES
GLIAL
NERVE SHEATH

AIDS AND CNS

H.I.V.INFECTION
     ACUTE
     CHRONIC PROGRESSIVE (AIDS RELATED
                      DEMENTIA)
OPPORTUNISTIC INFECTIONS

TUMORS

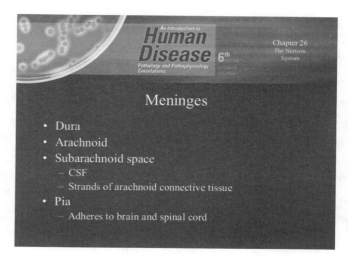

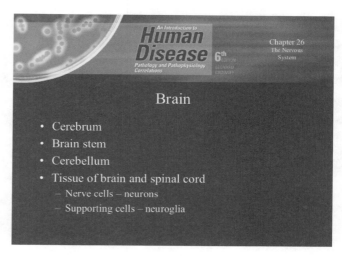

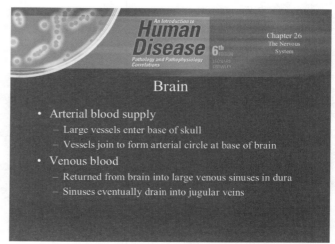

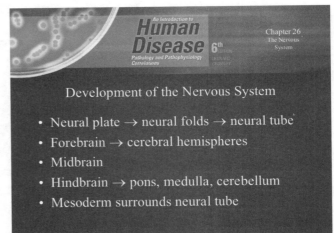

Development of the Nervous System

- Neural plate → neural folds → neural tube
- Forebrain → cerebral hemispheres
- Midbrain
- Hindbrain → pons, medulla, cerebellum
- Mesoderm surrounds neural tube

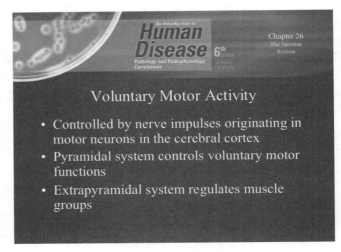

Voluntary Motor Activity

- Controlled by nerve impulses originating in motor neurons in the cerebral cortex
- Pyramidal system controls voluntary motor functions
- Extrapyramidal system regulates muscle groups

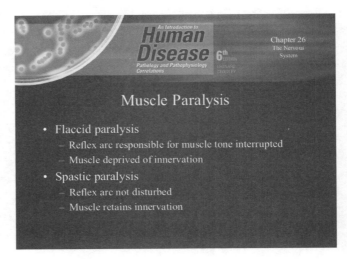

Muscle Paralysis

- Flaccid paralysis
  - Reflex arc responsible for muscle tone interrupted
  - Muscle deprived of innervation
- Spastic paralysis
  - Reflex arc not disturbed
  - Muscle retains innervation

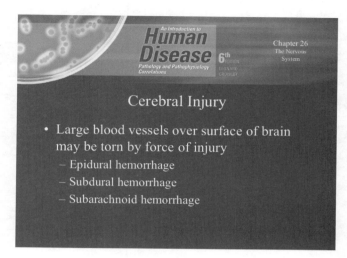

Cerebral Injury

- Large blood vessels over surface of brain may be torn by force of injury
  - Epidural hemorrhage
  - Subdural hemorrhage
  - Subarachnoid hemorrhage

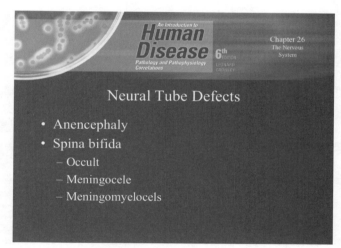

Neural Tube Defects

- Anencephaly
- Spina bifida
  - Occult
  - Meningocele
  - Meningomyelocels

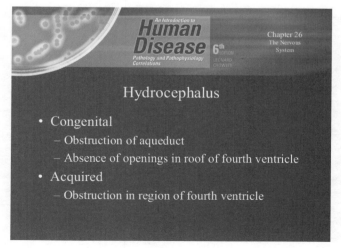

Hydrocephalus

- Congenital
  - Obstruction of aqueduct
  - Absence of openings in roof of fourth ventricle
- Acquired
  - Obstruction in region of fourth ventricle

Notes

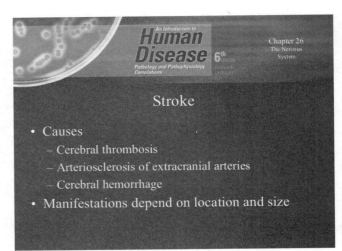

Stroke

- Causes
  - Cerebral thrombosis
  - Arteriosclerosis of extracranial arteries
  - Cerebral hemorrhage
- Manifestations depend on location and size

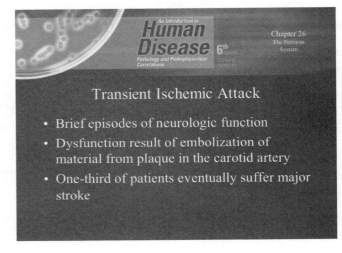

Transient Ischemic Attack

- Brief episodes of neurologic function
- Dysfunction result of embolization of material from plaque in the carotid artery
- One-third of patients eventually suffer major stroke

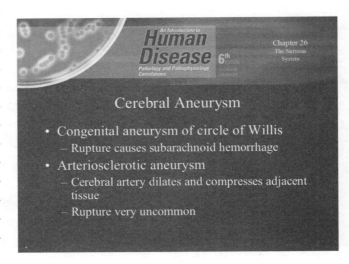

Cerebral Aneurysm

- Congenital aneurysm of circle of Willis
  - Rupture causes subarachnoid hemorrhage
- Arteriosclerotic aneurysm
  - Cerebral artery dilates and compresses adjacent tissue
  - Rupture very uncommon

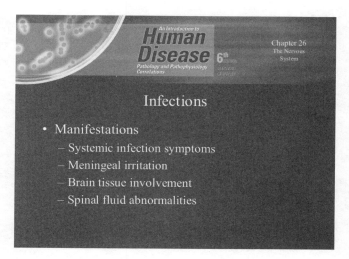

Infections

- Manifestations
  - Systemic infection symptoms
  - Meningeal irritation
  - Brain tissue involvement
  - Spinal fluid abnormalities

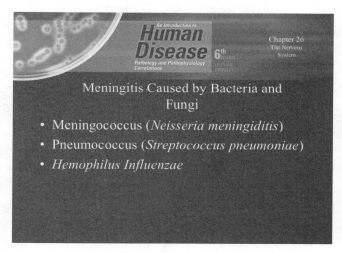

Meningitis Caused by Bacteria and Fungi

- Meningococcus (*Neisseria meningiditis*)
- Pneumococcus (*Streptococcus pneumoniae*)
- *Hemophilus Influenzae*

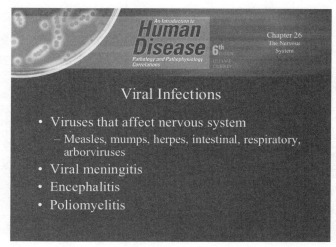

Viral Infections

- Viruses that affect nervous system
  - Measles, mumps, herpes, intestinal, respiratory, arborviruses
- Viral meningitis
- Encephalitis
- Poliomyelitis

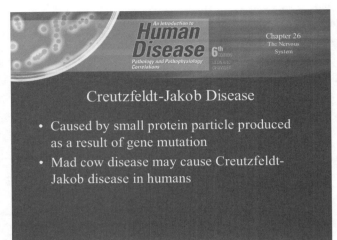

Creutzfeldt-Jakob Disease

- Caused by small protein particle produced as a result of gene mutation
- Mad cow disease may cause Creutzfeldt-Jakob disease in humans

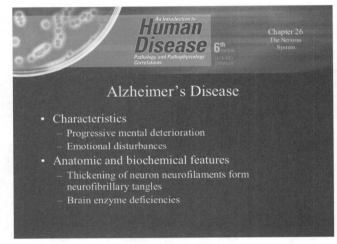

Alzheimer's Disease

- Characteristics
  - Progressive mental deterioration
  - Emotional disturbances
- Anatomic and biochemical features
  - Thickening of neuron neurofilaments form neurofibrillary tangles
  - Brain enzyme deficiencies

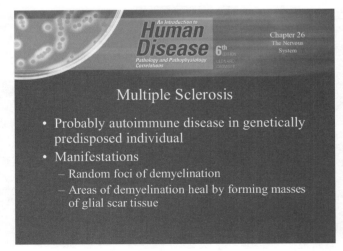

Multiple Sclerosis

- Probably autoimmune disease in genetically predisposed individual
- Manifestations
  - Random foci of demyelination
  - Areas of demyelination heal by forming masses of glial scar tissue

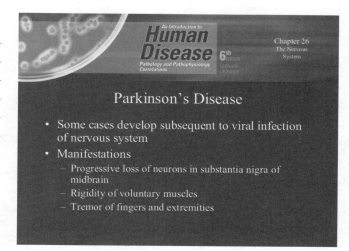

Parkinson's Disease

- Some cases develop subsequent to viral infection of nervous system
- Manifestations
  - Progressive loss of neurons in substantia nigra of midbrain
  - Rigidity of voluntary muscles
  - Tremor of fingers and extremities

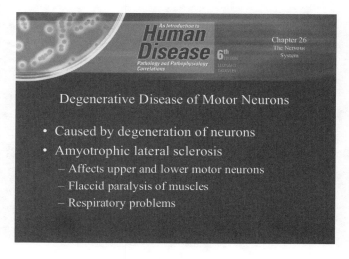

Degenerative Disease of Motor Neurons

- Caused by degeneration of neurons
- Amyotrophic lateral sclerosis
  - Affects upper and lower motor neurons
  - Flaccid paralysis of muscles
  - Respiratory problems

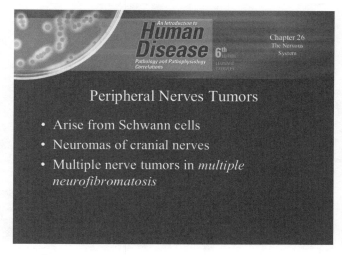

Peripheral Nerves Tumors

- Arise from Schwann cells
- Neuromas of cranial nerves
- Multiple nerve tumors in *multiple neurofibromatosis*

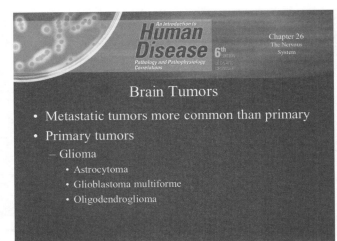

Brain Tumors

- Metastatic tumors more common than primary
- Primary tumors
  - Glioma
    - Astrocytoma
    - Glioblastoma multiforme
    - Oligodendroglioma

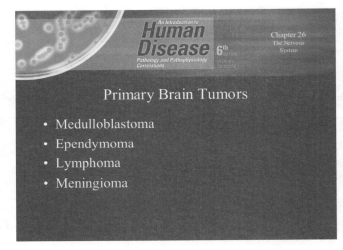

Primary Brain Tumors

- Medulloblastoma
- Ependymoma
- Lymphoma
- Meningioma

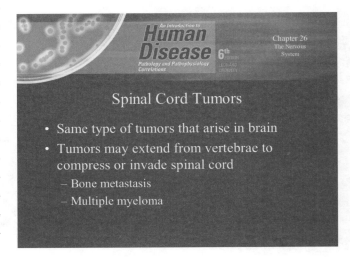

Spinal Cord Tumors

- Same type of tumors that arise in brain
- Tumors may extend from vertebrae to compress or invade spinal cord
  - Bone metastasis
  - Multiple myeloma

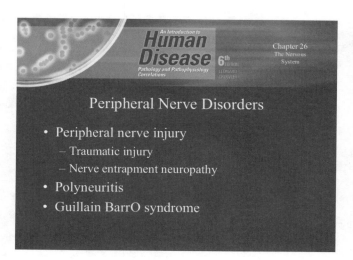

Peripheral Nerve Disorders

- Peripheral nerve injury
  - Traumatic injury
  - Nerve entrapment neuropathy
- Polyneuritis
- Guillain BarrO syndrome

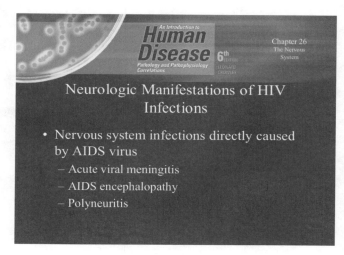

Neurologic Manifestations of HIV Infections

- Nervous system infections directly caused by AIDS virus
  - Acute viral meningitis
  - AIDS encephalopathy
  - Polyneuritis

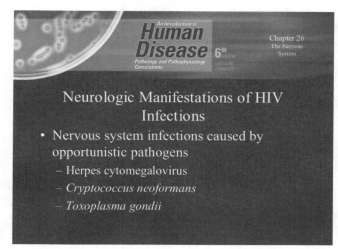

Neurologic Manifestations of HIV Infections

- Nervous system infections caused by opportunistic pathogens
  - Herpes cytomegalovirus
  - *Cryptococcus neoformans*
  - *Toxoplasma gondii*

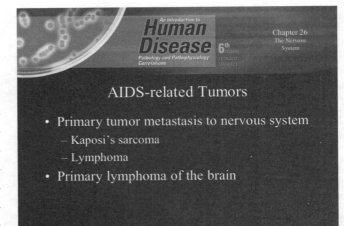

AIDS-related Tumors

- Primary tumor metastasis to nervous system
  - Kaposi's sarcoma
  - Lymphoma
- Primary lymphoma of the brain

Chapter Outline

The chapter outline provides you with an organizational guide to the topics and ideas presented in this chapter of the text.

Structure and Function of the Skeletal System
> Bone Formation
> Bone Growth

Congenital Malformations
> Abnormal Bone Formation
> Malformation of Fingers and Toes
> Congenital Clubfoot (Talipes)
> Congenital Dislocation of the Hip

Arthritis
> Rheumatoid Arthritis
> Osteoarthritis
> Gout

Fracture

Osteomyelitis
> Hematogenous Osteomyelitis
> Osteomyelitis as a Result of Direct Implantation of Bacteria
> Clinical Manifestations and Treatment

Tumors of Bone

Osteoporosis

Avascular Necrosis

Structure and Function of the Spine

Scoliosis

Intervertebral Disk Disease

Structure and Function of Skeletal Muscle
> Contraction of Skeletal Muscle
> Factors Affecting Muscular Structure and Function

Inflammation of Muscle (Myositis)
> Localized Myositis
> Generalized Myositis

Muscular Atrophy and Muscular Dystrophy

Myasthenia Gravis

Study Questions

The following questions are provided as a test for comprehension and as a study guide for use with the text chapters. Additional study material is located at http://health.jbpub.com/humandisease/, which contains useful eLearning tools such as an A&P review, animated flashcards, interactive online glossary, crossword puzzles, and Web links.

Key Terms

Define the following terms:

1. Endochondral bone formation _____

2. Fracture _____

3. Intervertebral disks _____

4. Rheumatoid arthritis _____

Fill-in-the-Blank

1. In a long bone, the thick tubular part is called the _____, and the end is called the _____.

2. The active bone-forming cells are called _____. The mature cells that become incorporated in the bone as it forms are called _____, and the large multinucleated cells that are concerned with bone resorption are called _____.

3. In a movable joint, the ends of the bones forming the joint are covered by _____ and the interior of the joint is lined by _____, which secretes _____ to lubricate the joint.

4. The two types of bone formation are called _____ bone formation, and _____ bone formation.

5. The hereditary condition characterized by disturbed endochondral bone formation that leads to a type of dwarfism in which the limbs are disproportionately short in relation to the trunk is called _____.

6. The congenital abnormality characterized by very thin, delicate bones that are easily broken under very minimal stress is called _____.

7. The name of the congenital condition in which the foot is turned inward on the ankle is called _____.

8. The inflammatory change in rheumatoid arthritis involves _____ initially, followed by spread of the inflammatory process over the surface of the joint.

9. A fracture in which the bone is broken into several fragments is called a _____ fracture.

10. A fracture in which the overlying skin is disrupted is called a _____ fracture.

11. The parts of the intervertebral disks are the _____ and the _____.

12. The condition characterized by a lateral curvature of the spine is called _____.

13. A systemic (collagen) disease characterized by inflammation of muscles and overlying skin is called _____.

14. A disease characterized by atrophy of muscles resulting from degeneration of the nerve cells supplying the muscles is called _____.

15. A disease characterized by atrophy and degeneration of muscles caused by abnormalities in the muscle fibers is called _____.

16. The autoimmune disease characterized by muscle weakness that is caused by progressive autoantibody-mediated damage to acetylcholine receptors at the myoneural junction of the muscle fiber is called

_____.

17. The two forms of muscular dystrophy are type _____ and type _____. The method of inheritance is _____. Sometimes the muscles of affected patients appear large because the muscle fibers have been replaced by _____.

True/False

Tell whether each statement is true or false. If false, explain why the statement is incorrect.

1. The blood and synovial tissues of rheumatoid arthritis (RA) patients contain an autoantibody directed against the patients' own gamma globulin. _____

_____

2. Immune complexes composed of gamma globulin and autoantibody are deposited in joints of RA patients.

_____

3. Antigen–antibody complexes activate complement and generate an inflammation within the joints in RA patients. _____

_____

4. Lymphocytes and macrophages attracted to the joints by the RA inflammatory process secrete cytokines (tumor necrosis factor) that damages joints. _____

_____

5. Drugs that block the effects of tumor necrosis factor have not been useful or effective in treating RA patients.

_____

Identify

1. Construct a table comparing the three main types of arthritis. (*Hint:* See Table 27-1.)

Characteristics	Rheumatoid Arthritis	Osteoarthritis	Gout

Matching

Match the types of arthritis on the right with each disease characteristic on the left.

1. _____ Affects primarily small bones of hands and feet   A. Osteoarthritis

2. _____ Autoantibodies formed   B. Rheumatoid arthritis

3. _____ Disturbed purine metabolism   C. Gout

4. _____ Major weight-bearing joints involved

5. _____ Fragmentation and degeneration of articular cartilage

6. _____ Destructive cytokines produced by inflammatory cells

7. _____ Uric acid deposit in an around joints

8. _____ May lead to kidney damage

Discussion Questions

1. What is a "slipped disk"? Why does it occur? Why does it sometimes produce pain radiating down the leg? How is it treated? _____

   _____

   _____

   _____

2. Explain whether each of the following descriptors applies to rheumatoid arthritis.

   a. Primarily a degenerative change involving major weight-bearing joints _____

   _____

   b. Deformities result from joint instability caused by destruction of articular surfaces or joints _____

   _____

   c. Associated with autoantibodies _____

   _____

   d. Involves the synovial linings _____

   _____

   e. Responds to antibiotic therapy _____

   _____

3. List the features that characterize gout. _____

   _____

   _____

   _____

4. What neoplastic processes may involve bone? _____

_____

_____

_____

5. What disease or condition affecting the skeletal system is due primarily to endocrine gland dysfunction?

_____

_____

_____

6. What is a herniated intervertebral disk? How does it occur? How is it detected? _____

_____

_____

_____

7. What is osteoporosis? What is the cause? How can it be prevented? _____

_____

_____

_____

BONES AND JOINTS

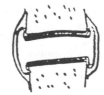

BURSAS
LIGAMENTS   MENISCI ETC.

OSTEOARTHRITIS (HYPERTROPHIC ARTHRITIS)

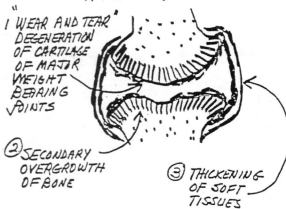

1 "WEAR AND TEAR" DEGENERATION OF CARTILAGE OF MAJOR WEIGHT BEARING JOINTS

② SECONDARY OVERGROWTH OF BONE

③ THICKENING OF SOFT TISSUES

RHEUMATOID ARTHRITIS

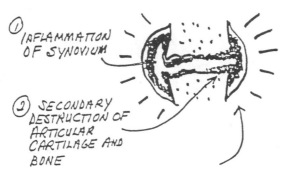

① INFLAMMATION OF SYNOVIUM

② SECONDARY DESTRUCTION OF ARTICULAR CARTILAGE AND BONE

③ DESTRUCTION OF JOINT SPACE
- INSTABILITY
- DEFORMATIES
- ANKYLOSIS

GOUT

1. DEPOSITION OF URIC ACID IN JOINT AND SYNOVIAL TISSUES

2. SECONDARY DAMAGE TO ARTICULAR TISSUES

③ SYSTEMIC EFFECTS
- TOPHI
- RENAL INJURY
- STONES

CLASSIFICATION
PRIMARY GOUT
SECONDARY GOUT

OSTEOPOROSIS

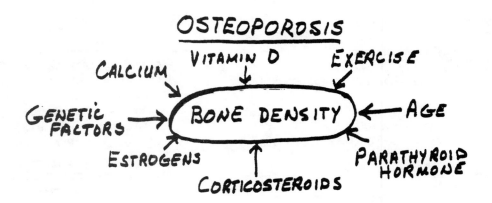

MANAGEMENT
  DIET AND EXERCISE
  1500 mg CA + VITAMIN D
  LIFE STYLE MODIFICATION: ALCOHOL. SMOKING

DRUGS FOR OSTEOPOROSIS

ESTROGEN

ESTROGENS: EFFECTIVE BUT NOT USED
  100 WOMEN GIVEN PRESCRIPTION
   20 NEVER FILL PRESCRIPTION
   50 DISCONTINUE WITHIN 1 YEAR
   30 CONTINUE

ALENDRONATE (BISPHOSPHONATE) INHIBITS
OSTEOCLASTS. GIVE WITH CALCIUM.
INCREASE BONE SPINE DENSITY 5% FIRST
YEAR AND THEN 1.5% PER YA
COMPARABLE INCREASE IN FEMORAL NECK
AND TROCHANTER DENSITY

CALCITONIN NASAL SPRAY INHIBITS
OSTEOCLASTS

SLOW RELEASE SODIUM FLUORIDE STIMULATES
OSTEOBLASTS (BUT TOO MUCH INCREASES
BONE FRAGILITY). GIVE WITH CALCIUM.
AND VITAMIN D.

TUMORS

PRIMARY: UNCOMMON
METASTATIC: COMMON

HERNIATED DISK:

NUCLEUS PROTRUDES
THROUGH WEAK AREA
IN ANNULUS AND
IMPINGES ON NERVE ROOTS

FRACTURES

SIMPLE   COMPOUND
COMMINUTED PATHOLOGIC

PARKINSON'S DISEASE

AN EXTRAPYRAMIDAL SYSTEM DISEASE
PYRAMIDAL: VOLUNTARY MOTOR ACTIVITY
EXTRAPYRAMIDAL: REGULATION · COORDINATION
BALANCE · POSTURE

MANIFESTATIONS
RIGIDITY · SLOW REDUCED MOVEMENTS ·
REST TREMOR · POSTURAL INSTABILITY

PATHOGENESIS
- NEURON LOSS IN SUBSTANTIA NIGRA.
- AXONS PROJECT TO BASAL GANGLIA AND LIBERATE DOPAMINE NEUROTRANSMITTER
- CONCENTRATION DOPAMINE FALLS IN BASAL GANGLIA

CAUSES
- IDIOPATHIC
- POST · ENCEPHALITIS
- DRUGS AND POISONS: MN, CO. STREET DRUGS
- TRANQUILIZERS AND ANTIPSYCHOTIC DRUGS THAT BLOCK DOPAMINE RECEPTORS IN CNS (REVERSIBLE)

TREATMENT
- L · DOPA (+ CARBIDOPA)
- DOPAMINE RECEPTOR AGONIST (BROMOCRIPTINE)
- ANTICHOLINERGIC DRUGS

MUSCLE FUNCTION DISORDERS

INVOLVING MOTOR NEURON
INVOLVING TRANSMISSION FROM NERVE TO MUSCLE
INVOLVING MUSCLE FIBER

MOTOR UNIT: ANT. HORN CELL AND ITS AXON, AND THE MUSCLE FIBERS IT INNERVATES

ANT HORN CELL (LOWER MOTOR NEURON)
CAN BE ACTIVATED BY
- SENSORY INPUT = REFLEX ARC
- CORTICAL NEURON (UPPER MOTOR NEURON) WITH AXON TRAVELLING IN CORTICOSPINAL (PYRAMIDAL TRACT) = VOLUNTARY MOTOR ACTIVITY

LOSS OF UPPER MOTOR NEURON = LOSS OF VOLUNTARY CONTROL · REFLEX FUNCTION AND MUSCLE TONE PRESERVED

LOSS OF LOWER MOTOR NEURON = NO MUSCLE FIBER INNERVATION. NO REFLEX ACTIVITY. NO MUSCLE TONE. PROFOUND MUSCLE ATROPHY.

DISEASES OF UPPER (CORTICAL) AND LOWER (BULBAR AND/OR SPINAL) NEURONS

AMYOTROPHIC LATERAL SCLEROSIS (ALS) AKA LOU GEHRIG'S DISEASE

MUSCULAR WEAKNESS · ATROPHY (LOWER MOTOR NEURONS · SPINAL CORD)

DIFFICULTY SWALLOWING AND TALKING (LOWER MOTOR NEURONS · BRAIN STEM)

MUSCULAR SPASTICITY · ABNORMAL REFLEXES (UPPER MOTOR NEURONS)

NO SENSORY DEFICIT
NO HEREDITARY PATTERN

DISEASE OF LOWER (BULBAR AND/OR SPINAL NEURONS ONLY
VARIOUS TYPES
VARIOUS MUSCLE GROUPS INVOLVED
VARIOUS AGES OF ONSET
VARIOUS INHERITANCE PATTERNS

CHILDHOOD TYPES
ADULT ONSET: PROGRESSIVE MUSCULAR ATROPHY

DISEASE OF MUSCLE FIBERS = MUSCULAR DYSTROPHY

DUCHENNE AND BECKER MUSC. DYSTROPHY

X LINKED HEREDITARY
GENE CODES FOR MUSCLE PROTEIN DYSTROPHIN REQUIRED FOR MUSCLE FUNCTION

DUCHENNE
DYSTROPHIN ABSENT
EARLY ONSET · RAPID PROGRESSION
MUSCLES MAY APPEAR HYPERTROPHIED
BECKER
ABNORMAL OR INSUFFICIENT DYSTROPHIN
LESS SEVERE · SLOWER PROGRESSION

DISEASE OF ACETYLCHOLINE RECEPTORS AT MYONEURAL JUNCTION = MYASTHENIA GRAVIS

AN AUTOIMMUNE DISEASE WITH ANTIBODY DIRECTED AGAINST ACETYLCHOLINE RECEPTORS

ABNORMAL FATIGUE OF VOLUNTARY MUSCLES

TREATED BY DRUGS THAT PROLONG ACTION OF ACETYLCHOLINE.

FACTORS INFLUENCING BONE DENSITY

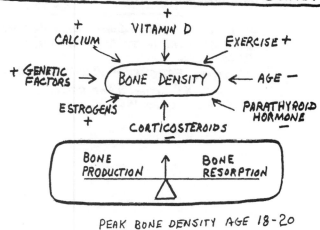

PEAK BONE DENSITY AGE 18-20

MANAGEMENT OF OSTEOPOROSIS

DIET AND WEIGHT BEARING EXERCISE
1500 MG CALCIUM + VITAMIN D
LIFE STYLE MODIFICATION:
    LIMIT ALCOHOL INTAKE
    NO SMOKING
ROUTINE BONE DENSITY SCREENING

DRUGS

- ESTROGENS, OR SELECTIVE ESTROGEN RECEPTOR MODULATORS
- BISPHOSPHONATES (ALENDRONATE) INCORPORATED IN BONE. INHIBITS OSTEOCLASTS.
- CALCITONIN NASAL SPRAY. INHIBITS OSTEOCLASTS
- (LOW DOSE PARATHYROID HORMONE) STIMULATES OSTEOBLASTS BUT NOT ENOUGH TO ALSO STIMULATE OSTEOCLASTS.

HERNIATED DISK

STRUCTURE AND FUNCTION OF DISKS

PATHOGENESIS
    NUCLEUS PULPOSUS PROTRUDES THROUGH WEAK AREA IN ANNULUS AND IMPINGES ON NERVE ROOTS EXITING THROUGH INTERVERTEBRAL FORAMEN
    PROTRUSION POSTEROLATERAL

TREATMENT
    CONSERVATIVE
    SURGICAL

SCOLIOSIS

MOST CASES IDIOPATHIC
EQUAL SEX INCIDENCE BUT PROGRESSION MORE COMMON IN GIRLS
PERSONS AT RISK: YOUNG PERSON WITH LARGE CURVE
MAYO RECOMMENDATIONS
(MAYO CLINIC PROC. 1995. 70: 978-82.
LESS THAN 20°: OBSERVATION - PERIODIC X RAYS
    20-40° BRACES
GREATER THAN 40° SURGERY (CAN ACHIEVE 50-75% CORRECTION

FRACTURES

SIMPLE
COMMINUTED
COMPOUND
PATHOLOGIC

TUMORS

METASTATIC - COMMON

PRIMARY - UNCOMMON
OF BONE - CARTILAGE
OF PLASMA CELLS IN MARROW (MYELOMA)

MUSCLE FUNCTION DISORDERS

(INVOLVING MOTOR NEURON)

    PROGRESSIVE MUSCULAR ATROPHY
    AMYOTROPHIC LATERAL SCLEROSIS
    PARKINSONS DISEASE

(INVOLVING TRANSMISSION FROM NERVE TO MUSCLE)

    MYASTHENIA GRAVIS

(INVOLVING MUSCLE FIBER)

    MUSCULAR DYSTROPHY

DISEASE OF ACETYLCHOLINE RECEPTORS
AT MYONEURAL JUNCTION = MYASTHENIA
GRAVIS

AN AUTOIMMUNE DISEASE WITH ANTIBODY
DIRECTED AGAINST ACETYLCHOLINE
RECEPTORS

ABNORMAL FATIGUE OF VOLUNTARY MUSCLES

TREATED BY DRUGS THAT PROLONG ACTION
OF ACETYLCHOLINE.

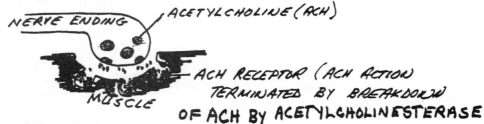

NERVE ENDING   ACETYLCHOLINE (ACH)

MUSCLE

ACH RECEPTOR (ACH ACTION
TERMINATED BY BREAKDOWN
OF ACH BY ACETYLCHOLINESTERASE

MANIFESTATIONS:
MUSCLE WEAKNESS
TREATMENT: DRUGS TO INHIBIT ACETYLCHOLINESTERASE
AND PROLONG ACH ACTION)

DISEASE OF MUSCLE FIBERS = MUSCULAR
DYSTROPHY

DUCHENNE AND BECKER MUSC. DYSTROPHY

  X LINKED HEREDITARY

  GENE CODES FOR MUSCLE PROTEIN DYSTROPHIN
    REQUIRED FOR MUSCLE FUNCTION

  DUCHENNE
    DYSTROPHIN ABSENT
    EARLY ONSET - RAPID PROGRESSION
    MUSCLES MAY APPEAR HYPERTROPHIED
  BECKER
    ABNORMAL OR INSUFFICIENT DYSTROPHIN
    LESS SEVERE SLOWER PROGRESSION

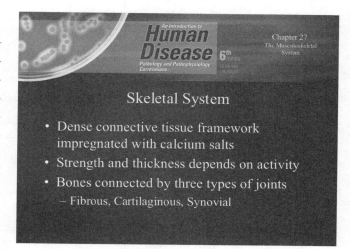

Skeletal System

- Dense connective tissue framework impregnated with calcium salts
- Strength and thickness depends on activity
- Bones connected by three types of joints
  - Fibrous, Cartilaginous, Synovial

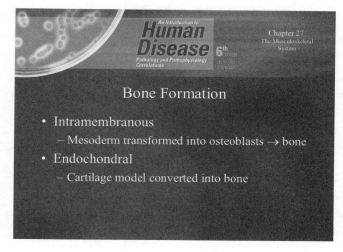

Bone Formation

- Intramembranous
  - Mesoderm transformed into osteoblasts → bone
- Endochondral
  - Cartilage model converted into bone

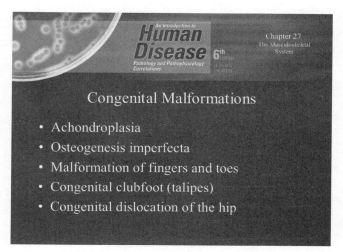

Congenital Malformations

- Achondroplasia
- Osteogenesis imperfecta
- Malformation of fingers and toes
- Congenital clubfoot (talipes)
- Congenital dislocation of the hip

Notes

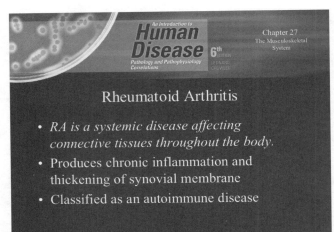

Rheumatoid Arthritis

- *RA is a systemic disease affecting connective tissues throughout the body.*
- Produces chronic inflammation and thickening of synovial membrane
- Classified as an autoimmune disease

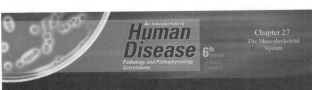

Osteoarthritis

- *Osteoarthritis is a "wear and tear" degeneration of one or more weight bearing joints.*
- Causes degenerative of articular cartilage
- Manifestation of normal aging process

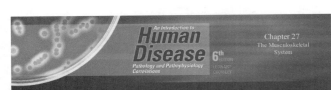

Gout

- Disorder of purine metabolism
- Acute episodes caused by precipitation of uric acid crystals in joint fluid
- Uric acid stones also may form within kidney and lower urinary tract

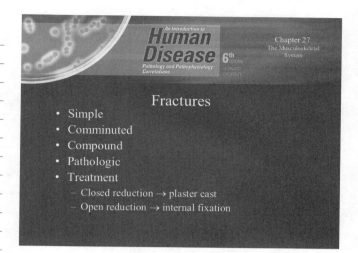

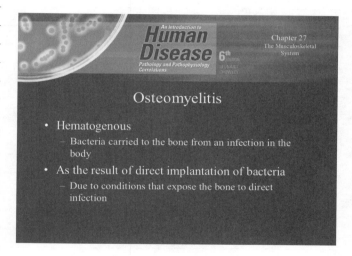

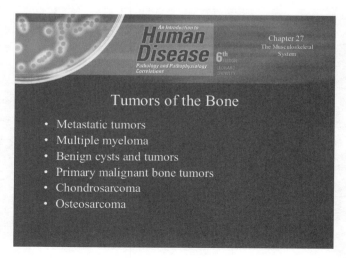

Notes

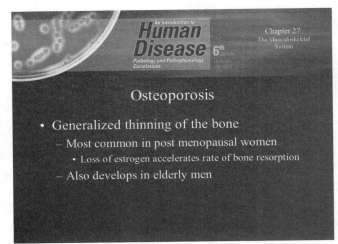

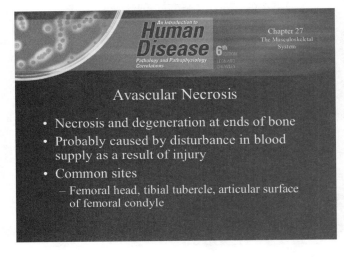

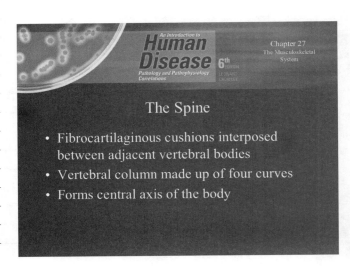

Notes

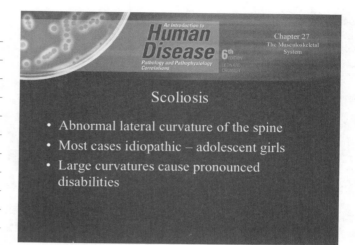

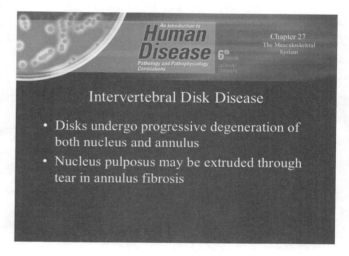

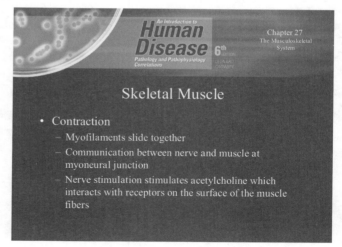

Notes

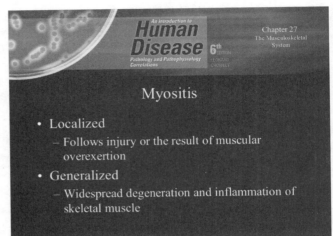

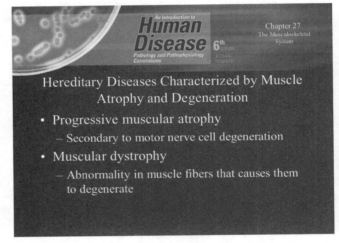

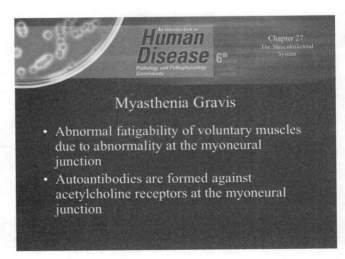